Pediatric Heart Sounds

Michael E. McConnell
with contributions by Alan Branigan

Pediatric Heart Sounds

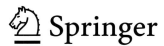 Springer

Michael E. McConnell, MD
Emory University and the Sibley Heart Center
Cardiology at 52 Executive Park South
Suite 5200.
Atlanta, GA 30329
USA

with contributions by
Alan Branigan, MA, MEd
Director, Educational Support
Eastern Area Health Education Center
2000 Venture Tower Dr.
Greenville, NC 27835-7224
USA

ISBN 978-1-84628-683-4   e-ISBN 978-1-84628-684-1
DOI 10.1007/978-1-84628-684-1

British Library Cataloguing in Publication Data
A catalogue record for this book is available from the British Library

Library of Congress Control Number: 2008931524

Printed on acid-free paper

Springer Science+Business Media
springer.com

Preface

Why another book to teach auscultation? Isn't the use of the stethoscope a "lost art", totally unnecessary in the age of echocardiography and "hand held" imaging "stethoscopes"? The answer is that there is perhaps no other physical examination skill that a physician making patient care decisions must have that is more important, even now. If a patient complains of fever and a cough, a chest radiograph interpreted by someone else will either confirm or rule out the diagnosis of pneumonia, and a quick look in a textbook can tell the physician the next course to take. When a patient comes to the office with no complaints, and on auscultation has a soft systolic murmur, only good physical examination skills will allow the examiner to reassure the patient that the murmur is non-pathologic. There is unfortunately ample evidence that auscultatory skills are very poorly taught to medical students and residents [1]. Research does show that intensive instruction, followed by reexamining patients with known lesions, will improve the diagnostic accuracy. Unfortunately, in busy practices, the ability of the learner to listen, discuss the findings with the preceptor, and to listen again is often lacking [2]. The inability to appreciate abnormalities of precordial activity, to critically listen to the first and second heart sounds, and to discern the difference between a pathologic murmur and a functional one often leads to unnecessary testing, and potentially leads to missed diagnoses.

There are ample sources to help improve physical examination skills, many written by the true great teachers of medicine. Yet, in spite of these, auscultation skills are poorly learned. With the advent of new "multimedia" technology, perhaps auscutation can be more effectively taught. Unfortunately, recent evidence with some multimedia teaching tools suggests that the learning is still ineffective [1]. The CD-ROM that accompanies this text uses a novel approach to educate the learner about auscultation skills. It is not meant to be an exhaustive "encyclopedia", listing every possible abnormal sound that the heart can make. The goal is to get the learner more comfortable using the stethoscope in an organized fashion, and once they have the organized system of auscultation, to improve their ability to tell pathologic from normal heart sounds. The cardiac sounds on the CD-ROM were recorded from patients with the specific cardiac abnormalities listed, and the specific pathology was confirmed using echocardiography. The programmed nature of the CD-ROM forces the learner to critically evaluate all aspects of the cardiac examination. By placing the findings in the spread sheet, and getting immediate feedback on correct and incorrect responses, the learner's ability to listen critically should improve.

References

1. Mahnke CB, Nowalk A, Hofkosh D, Zuberbuhler JR, Law YM (2004) Comparison of two educational interventions on pediatric resident auscultation skills. Pediatrics 113(5):1331–1335

2. Favrat B, Pecoud A, Jaussi A (2004) Teaching cardiac auscultation to trainees in internal medicine and family practice: does it work? BMC Med Educ 4(1):5

Contents

Contents

Chapter 1
Normal Heart Sounds

M.E. McConnell, *Pediatric Heart Sounds*,
DOI: 10.1007/978-1-84628-684-1_1, © Springer-Verlag London Limited 2008

The First Heart Sound

The normal heart makes many different normal sounds. Proper cardiac auscultation can only be accomplished if the listener concentrates on each cardiac sound individually. The listening areas are named for the valve that is best heard in that location. It does not mean that you cannot hear the other valves close, just that the valve the area is named for is best heard in that location (Fig. 1.1).

Listening to individual sounds and timing is known as listening with "dissection." Contraction of the ventricles is termed ventricular systole and is the time in the cardiac cycle when blood is ejected from the ventricles into the great vessels. At the beginning of ventricular systole, the mitral and tricuspid valves close, causing the first heart sound. Using the high-pitched side of the stethoscope, the diaphragm, and listening at the lower left sternal border, the first sound should be easily heard in patients with a normal heart

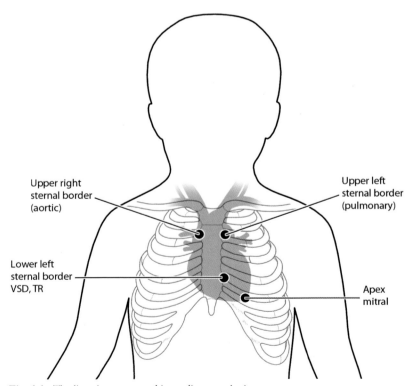

Upper right
sternal border
(aortic)

Upper left
sternal border
(pulmonary)

Lower left
sternal border
VSD, TR

Apex
mitral

Fig. 1.1. The listening areas used in cardiac auscultation

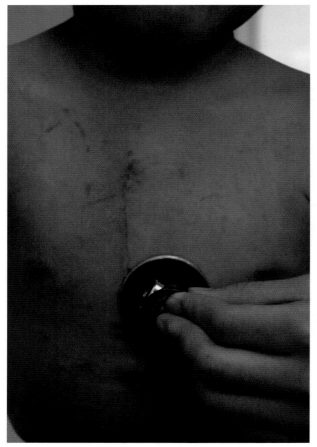

Fig. 1.2. Listening for the first heart sound. The diaphragm of the stethoscope is placed at the lower left sternal border (the tricuspid area)

(see Fig. 1.2). These valves usually close within 100 ms resulting in a first heart sound that sounds like a single sound [1]. It is easier to discern the first from the second heart sound at low heart rates. If it is unclear which sound is which, palpation of a brachial pulse during auscultation is useful. Because the closure of the mitral and tricuspid valves begins ventricular systole, the pulse should follow the first heart sound. Once the timing of the two heart sounds is clear, focusing on listening to each sound individually is easier.

Listen to the normal heart sound recording on the CD-ROM. The recording of the first heart sound is a very clear closure sound of the mitral and tricuspid valves. This first heart sound is also known

Table 1.1. What you hear on the CD-ROM

Normal heart sounds	Upper right sternal border	Upper left sternal border	Lower left sternal border	Apex
First heart sound	Not audible	Very soft	Low pitched thud, heard best at the lower left sternal border	Soft single sound
Second heart sound	Single	Splits with respiration	Slightly louder than S1, single	Single sound, slightly louder than S1
Systole	No murmur	No murmur	No murmur	No murmur
Diastole	No murmur	No murmur	No murmur	No murmur

as S1. It is lower pitched than the second heart sound (S2), but is still well heard at the lower left sternal border using the diaphragm of the stethoscope (Table 1.1).

If the first heart sound "slurs" or splits, this could be an indication of cardiac pathology. This slurring of the first heart sound may be caused by asynchronous closure of the mitral and tricuspid valves, and could be a normal finding. Other possibilities for the "splitting" of the first heart sound would include clicks. All four of the cardiac valves may make clicking sounds. Each of the clicks has differentiating characteristics that will be discussed below.

A split first heart sound that is heard best at the apex may be related to an abnormal aortic valve. After the mitral and tricuspid valves close, the abnormal aortic valve will open, making a clicking sound. A "split" first heart sound that is heard best at the apex or the upper right sternal border may be caused by an abnormal aortic valve. After the mitral and tricuspid valves close, the abnormal aortic valve will open, making a clicking sound. This type of "splitting" of the first heart sound is not a true "split" first heart sound. Rather the first heart sound, caused by the closure of the mitral and tricuspid valves precedes the aortic valve click [2]. With the stethoscope, the click sounds like a split first heart sound. For this reason, thinking of aortic valve clicks as a "split first heart sound heard best at the apex" is a simple way to remember when listening to a patient with an aortic valve click.

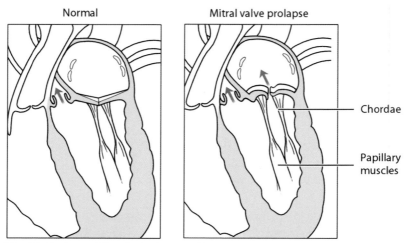

Fig. 1.3. Prolapse of the mitral valve caused by decreasing the intracardiac volume. This is done by having the patient stand while listening with the diaphragm at the apex (the mitral area)

The mitral valve click is best heard at the apex, and often while the patient is in the standing position. The prolapsing mitral valve may have more length to the combined length of the papillary muscle, chordae tendenae, and valve leaflets (see Fig. 1.3). This allows the mitral valve to prolapse into the left atrium, and may cause a clicking sound heard at the apex. Maneuvers that decrease the volume of the left ventricle, such as standing, will allow the mitral valve to prolapse more. Standing causes intravascular fluid to move into the lower extremities and the pelvis, leaving less blood to fill the heart. The mitral valve structures, such as the chordae and the valve leaflets, have a fixed length that does not change when the patient is in a standing position. If there is less blood in the heart, because of the patient standing and gravity taking blood down to the lower extremities, then the mitral valve will have more length relative to the size of the ventricle, and will possibly move above the mitral valve annulus with systole. When this happens, the mitral valve prolapses. This is why the click of mitral valve prolapse is best heard while the patient is standing.

Pulmonary valve clicks often sound like split first heart sounds, and are heard at the upper left sternal border (the pulmonic area) [3]. The clicking pulmonary valve also causes a "split" first heart sound, similar to the aortic click. The major difference is that the click of a pulmonary valve is heard at the upper left sternal border, and the sound changes with respiration. When the patient inhales, the negative intrathoracic pressure increases venous return to the right side of the heart. This augmented return causes the abnormal, clicking pulmonary valve to float superiorly, and the click becomes softer. The pulmonary ejection click often sounds like a split first heart sound that disappears when the patient takes in a breath. Occasionally pulmonary valve ejection clicks are so loud that they are palpable at the upper left sternal border, and the click can still disappear with inspiration.

The last of the four cardiac valves that can click, and therefore alter the first heart sound, is the tricuspid valve. Tricuspid valves can often be significantly deformed in apparently healthy patients, specifically those with less severe variants of Ebstein anomaly. In Ebstein anomaly, the abnormal tricuspid valve is positioned toward the apex of the right ventricle. The abnormal valve may billow with systole, causing multiple systolic clicks.

Another abnormality of the first heart sound that indicates cardiac pathology is if the first heart sound is inaudible at the lower left sternal border. This is occasionally due to morbid obesity in an older child, but usually is related to abnormal cardiac sounds that cover up, or obscure the closure of the mitral and tricuspid valves. These abnormalities include ventricular septal defects, patent arterial ducts, some forms of mitral or tricuspid valve regurgitation, and lastly severe right ventricular outflow tract obstruction. All of these causes of murmurs that obscure the first heart sound are pathologic, and therefore would require that the child have an evaluation by a pediatric cardiologist. Therefore, listening for the presence or absence of the first heart sound at the lower left sternal border can often be a "quick study" to help differentiate a functional (innocent or normal) murmur from a murmur caused by cardiac pathology. If the listener cannot hear the closure of the mitral and tricuspid valves because the sound is obscured by a murmur, it is likely that the child will have some type of congenital heart disease.

In summary, the first heart sound is a high-pitched sound best heard with the diaphragm of the stethoscope, and best heard at the lower left sternal border. Splitting of the first hears sound may be heard in patients with asynchronous closure of the mitral and tricuspid valves, and therefore the splitting of S1 may be a variant of normal. "Splitting" of the first heart sound may also indicate cardiac pathology, caused by aortic, mitral, tricuspid, or pulmonary valve abnormalities. If you cannot hear the closure of the mitral and tricuspid valves because the first heart sound is obscured by a murmur, the patient is quite likely to have cardiac pathology

The Second Heart Sound

After listening carefully for the first heart sound at the lower left sternal border, the listener should then move the diaphragm of the stethoscope to the upper left sternal border and listen to the second heart sound (S2) (Fig. 1.4). Many cardiologists consider the second heart sound to be the most important component of cardiac auscultation. It is very important to understand what causes this sound, and also what causes the changes in the second heart sound during the respiratory cycle. This is necessary in order to more easily understand the cardiac auscultatory findings of different cardiac lesions, as will be discussed later in this book, and heard on the CD. The upper left sternal border is the best location to hear the closure sound of the pulmonic valve, as well as the aortic valve. Together these two closure sounds make up the second heart sound, or S2. The two semilunar valves close simultaneously during exhalation, and a single sound is audible.

When the patient inhales, the increased venous return to the right side of the heart brings more blood into the right ventricle. The ejection of this increased volume of blood takes longer than the left ventricular ejection, and therefore the pulmonary valve closes after the aortic valve. The splitting of the second heart sound is related not only to the increased venous return, but also to the pressures in the aorta and pulmonary artery. The aortic pressure is significantly higher than the pulmonary artery pressure. The pressure in the aorta in diastole is reflected in the blood pressure, and varies with age. The aortic diastolic pressure is usually within 40 and 80 mmHg. The pulmonary artery diastolic pressure is much lower than the aortic pressure, and is generally between 5 and 15 mmHg. Ordinarily this splitting of the second heart sound is 40 ms or less in normal children. The pulmonary valve is anterior to the aortic valve, and

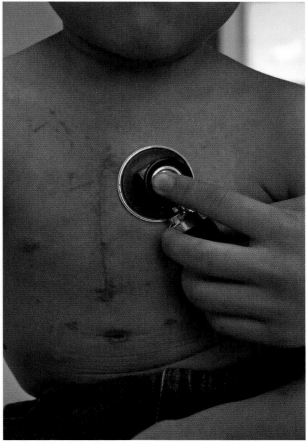

Fig. 1.4. The stethoscope position at the upper left sternal border. This is the best location to hear the splitting of the second heart sound

is therefore directly beneath the sternum in a patient with a normal heart. When the patient takes in a breath, the second heart sound splits, and both components of the second heart sound have similar intensity.

Of course, a small child is unlikely to take a deep breath and hold it, so the listener must gain proficiency at listening to hearts with rapid heart rates in uncooperative patients. By concentrating on the second heart sound at the upper left sternal border, the listener should eventually appreciate that the second heart sound is not constant, and that it changes (even if it is slightly). This means that the pulmonary valve closes after the aortic valve.

If the second heart sound is always split, it means that the pulmonary valve always closes after the aortic valve. There are two common explanations for this physical finding. The first is a cardiac electrical abnormality, specifically complete right bundle branch block (Fig. 1.5). This is often a post-operative phenomenon seen in patients who had surgical closure of a ventricular septal defect. The other explanation, and the reason why I would encourage the reader of this book to pay particular attention to the second heart sound, is that widely split second heart sounds are heard in patients with hemodynamically significant atrial septal defects. Remember that the inspiration brings more blood into the right ventricle. In patients with atrial septal defects, because of the left to right shunt at the atrial level, the right side of the circulation always has additional blood, just as if the patient always took in a deep breath. The result is that the second heart sound acts at all times like the patient took in a deep breath, and it is always split.

A loud single second heart sound that does not vary with respiration indicates cardiac pathology. It is heard in patients with pulmonary artery hypertension because the pressure closing the aortic and pulmonic valves is the same. The semilunar valves therefore close at the same time and with equal intensity. Ordinarily, the pulmonary artery pressure is much lower than the aortic pressure,

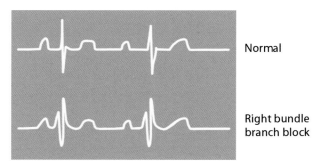

Normal

Right bundle
branch block

Fig. 1.5. Complete right bundle branch block recorded in V1 in comparison to a normal EKG. The wide QRS complex means that the electrical impulse moves slowly through the myocardium, and the right ventricle depolarizes after the left, causing the right ventricle to eject its contents after the left ventricle. The pulmonary valve therefore closes after the aortic valve, giving a "fixed split"

and the pressure closing the pulmonary valve is therefore much lower. The pulmonary valve is anterior to the aorta, so even if the sound is lower in intensity, it is well heard. If, for example, the patient has pulmonary hypertension, the pressure closing the pulmonary valve causes the anterior semilunar valve to close early, resulting in a loud single second heart sound. Some forms of congenital heart disease have malposition of the great vessels so that the aorta is anterior to the pulmonary valve. These patients also have loud single second heart sounds because the closure sound of the anterior aorta overwhelms the closure of the posterior pulmonary artery.

Paying particular attention to the second heart sound is possibly the most important part of the cardiac physical examination. Variable splitting of S2 tells that the patient has two semilunar valves, that the pressure in the pulmonary artery is lower than the aortic pressure, and that the contents of the right ventricle vary with respiration. This is a great deal of information about the cardiovascular system that is gleaned from listening carefully to an isolated part of the chest!

Now please take time to listen to the CD-ROM, beginning with the normal heart sounds. Move the virtual stethoscope to the lower left sternal border, and listen to the first heart sound. When you are confident you can hear this sound separately from the second heart sound, move the stethoscope to the upper left sternal border and concentrate on the second heart sound. Listen carefully, and convince yourself that the sound is not constant, and that it changes with respiration. If you cannot convince yourself that the second heart sound splits or changes with respiration, go to the ventricular septal defect recording. In this recording, at the upper left sternal border (the pulmonic area), the second heart sound is well heard, and it splits every other beat. (This is because the child that this recording came from was so uncooperative that only two cardiac cycles of the recording were usable: one with inspiration and one during exhalation.) Once the listener gets the "rhythm" of the splitting, it becomes more obvious. Remember, no one was born with these skills, so with work and attention to details such as the first and second heart sounds, you can improve your auscultatory skills.

References

1. Nadas A (1957) Pediatric cardiology. WB Saunders, Philadelphia

2. Leatham A (1951) Phonocardiogram of aortic stenosis. Br Heart J 13:153.

3. Leatham A, Vogelpool L (1954) The early systolic sound in dilatation of the pulmonary artery. Br Heart J 16:21

Chapter 2
Innocent Heart Murmurs

M.E. McConnell, *Pediatric Heart Sounds*,
DOI: 10.1007/978-1-84628-684-1_2, © Springer-Verlag London Limited 2008

Innocent Murmurs

Almost every child you listen to with a stethoscope will have a heart murmur. The incidence of congenital heart disease is approximately 8 per 1,000, so this means that the vast majority of children with heart murmurs have a normal heart. The aim of this book is to get you more comfortable not only hearing murmurs but also being able to tell a "normal" murmur from a pathologic one. The presence or absence of a murmur cannot be the reason for referral, either to a cardiologist, or worse yet, to an echo machine. The latter approach has been shown to be a very cost-ineffective way to evaluate heart murmurs [1]. The reason is that 80% of normal children have a murmur and roughly 1% has structural heart disease. You will order roughly 80,000 dollars worth of echocardiograms (in 2005 US dollars) for every child who has heart disease, and that is not taking into account that the etiology of the murmur may be missed on echocardiography [2]. The hope is that the reader of this book (and when used in conjunction with the CD-ROM) will be able to determine if the murmur is likely to be pathologic or functional; therefore, increasing the likelihood that whether a referral to a pediatric cardiologist is necessary. Remember, the presence or absence of a murmur is not the reason a patient should be referred to a pediatric cardiologist. Normal murmurs are also known as functional or innocent murmurs. This means that if the heart ejects its contents, a noise is made. The list of functional murmurs includes seven possibilities, as reviewed in the excellent article by Pelech et al. [3]. Because three of these murmurs are by far the most common, in the interest of simplicity, they will be discussed individually in detail. The three common innocent or functional murmurs are peripheral pulmonary "stenosis," a Still's murmur, and the adolescent outflow murmur. All are normal, and the patients have normal heart and do not require a special medication.

Peripheral Pulmonary Flow Murmurs

Peripheral pulmonary stenosis murmurs commonly present by 6 weeks of age and usually resolve by 1 year of age. They are very common and are not associated with long-term pathologic consequences. In order to understand the peripheral pulmonary "stenosis" murmur, it is important to understand a little about the fetal circulation.

Fetal blood flow is very different from a normal adult circulation (see Fig. 2.1). The fetus has two communications between the right and left sides of the circulation, the atrial septal defect, and the patent arterial duct. These communications allow the oxygenated blood in the fetus to get to the most vital organ, the brain. The communication also results in the most desaturated blood (meaning the blood with the least oxygen) going to the oxygen source (the placenta). The circulation is as follows: the red blood cell that has just passed through the placenta now has increased oxygen, since the placenta functions as the infant's oxygen source. The cell flows into the inferior vena cava through the venous duct. When it gets to the heart, the Eustachian valve baffles this blood to the left atrium

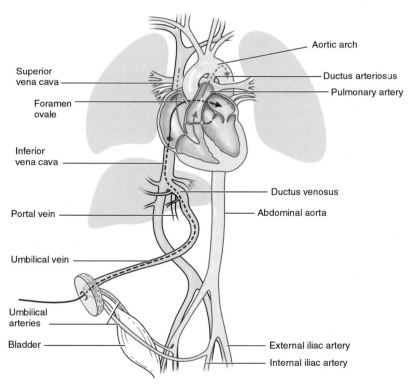

Fig. 2.1. The fetal circulation. Note the presence of an intracardiac shunt in the atrial septum, and the extra cardiac shunt at the arterial duct. See text for details

through the hole in the atrial septum called the ostium secundum. This means that the most oxygenated blood in the fetus is now in the left atrium where it goes through the mitral valve to the left ventricle, then to the aorta, and up to the fetus' developing brain. The brain extracts oxygen from the blood, and then the blood returns to the superior vena cava and then to the right atrium. The brain extracts a great deal of oxygen from the red blood cells, and now the red blood cell is "desaturated." The cell then flows from the superior vena cava to the right atrium, through the tricuspid valve, and into the right ventricle where it is pumped out to the pulmonary artery. Now the blood cell has three possible paths. It could go to the right lung via the right pulmonary artery, to the left lung via the left pulmonary artery, or to the arterial duct and into the descending aorta. Because the lungs are not inflated, there is no reason for much blood flow to pass into either the right or left pulmonary artery. Most of the blood ejected by the right ventricle goes through the arterial duct and into the descending aorta. This desaturated blood perfuses either the fetus' lower body or the placenta. Because of the limited blood flow to the lungs, the pulmonary arteries in the newborn are small [4]. The relatively small pulmonary arteries play a part in the peripheral pulmonary flow murmur.

At birth, multiple changes take place. The infant takes a deep breath, opening the lungs, and shortly after birth the arterial duct, the venous duct, and the secundum atrial defect should close. The pulmonary blood flow then increases from less than 10% of the fetus' cardiac output to 100% of the cardiac output.

The other changing event in newborns deals with the hematocrit. The newborn has a very high hematocrit because in the uterus the oxygen saturation level in the blood stream for the most highly oxygenated blood is only 80–90%. Therefore, the fetus needs an increased number of red blood cells to transport oxygen adequately. After birth, the oxygen saturation should increase to nearly 100%, and subsequently the hemoglobin in the newborn infant will gradually decline from the as high as 19 g/dl at birth to 9 g/dl by 7–10 weeks of age (the so-called physiologic "nadir") [5]. So now there are two factors that cause many normal infants to have a murmur generated by blood flow into the lungs. First is the pulmonary arteries that had limited blood flow in the uterus, and are therefore small, and the second is the increasing cardiac output associated with the declining hemoglobin level. The peripheral pulmonary flow murmur is a common consequence of these two physiologic events in normal infants. The peripheral pulmonary stenosis murmur is the consequence of flow turbulence made by blood flowing from the right ventricle to the pulmonary arteries. The infant should be asymptomatic, feeding, and growing well. The precordial palpation is normal, and there should be no thrills or heaves. Because the sound of a peripheral pulmonary flow murmur begins after the ventricular contraction and therefore after the AV valve closes, the first heart sound caused by the closure of the mitral and tricuspid valve should be easily heard at the lower left sternal border. The pulmonary artery pressure should be normal in these infants; therefore, the second heart sound should also be normal. This means the second heart sound should split with inspiration. Because of the rapid heartbeat, it may be possible only to note that the second heart sound does not sound the same at all times. The murmur of peripheral pulmonary stenosis is heard best in the pulmonary area, and also radiates along the pulmonary arteries. What this means is that because the pulmonary arteries go to each lung, the murmur is often heard in the right and left lateral chest. There should be no diastolic murmur; therefore, the entire exam should be as noted in Table 2.1.

I would encourage pediatricians and family physicians caring for asymptomatic healthy infants with soft systolic ejection murmurs at the upper left sternal border as described above to reassure the parents and follow the patients without referral to a cardiologist.

Table 2.1. Peripheral pulmonary flow murmur

Precordial activity	Normal
First heart sound (S1)	Normal
Second heart sound (S2)	Normal (splits with respiration)
Systolic murmur	
Grade	Grade 1–3
Location	Left upper sternal border, often radiating to the axillae bilaterally
Diastolic murmur	None
Femoral pulses	Normal

These soft systolic murmurs are extremely common and should resolve by the time the child is about 12 months of age.

Referral of a child with this type of murmur to a pediatric cardiologist may result in the following scenario. A soft systolic murmur at the upper left sternal border may be because of the normal flow across relatively small pulmonary arteries (the peripheral pulmonary flow murmur) or could be caused by increased blood flow across normal pulmonary arteries. The pathologic cause of increased flow across normal pulmonary arteries would be an atrial septal defect (the physical examination for this will be discussed at length in its own section). Because even the most skilled pediatric cardiologist cannot tell the difference on physical examination between a peripheral pulmonary flow murmur and an atrial septal defect in all infants, the infant with a peripheral pulmonary flow murmur will often get an echocardiogram. Hopefully the echocardiogram will be normal, but often a small residual hole in the atrial septum is seen. This often results in a return appointment to the cardiologist and the need for a second echocardiogram. The better scenario is an asymptomatic child with a soft systolic murmur at the upper left sternal border would be followed by the pediatrician or family physician at routine child visits and the physician will hopefully note that the murmur resolves. If the patient does indeed have an atrial defect, the physical exam findings should become more obvious over time. There is no medical urgency to know if an asymptomatic child has a small defect in the atrial septum that is likely to close spontaneously. In summary, a peripheral pulmonary flow murmur is a soft systolic murmur often heard in asymptomatic infants. The murmur should resolve spontaneously and does not necessarily warrant referral to a pediatric cardiologist.

Still's Murmur

The second type of functional or innocent or normal murmur is the "Still's murmur." It was first described by Dr. Still in the early twentieth century, and is commonly heard for the first time in a child aged 3–6 years. Often parents are quite indignant that they have never been told their child had a murmur before, but the fact is that the child may not have had a murmur prior to the 3–6-year examination. The murmur is occasionally heard in infants, and may be present in adolescents. The exact etiology of a Still's murmur is unknown, but hypotheses include vibrations in either the right or left ventricle, or "tendons" often seen in the left ventricle [6]. Dr. Still described the murmur as "twanging," implying that the sound has musical qualities [7]. The Still's murmur is frequently lower pitched than other systolic murmurs, and hence is heard well with the "low-frequency" side of the stethoscope, the bell. Because the murmur is not pathologic, the precordial activity is normal, meaning there are no heaves (which would be caused by increased cardiac output), or thrills (caused by turbulent rapidly moving blood). The Still's murmur begins after the mitral and tricuspid valves close, meaning that S1 at the lower left sternal border is audible and normal. Because there is neither pulmonary hypertension nor increased pulmonary blood flow in patients with a Still's murmur, the second heart sound should be normal, splitting when the child inhales (Table 2.2).

There are two nuances associated with functional, innocent, or Still's murmurs that require understanding. The first is the concept of a "venous hum." In the interest of simplicity (remember this is not an encyclopedia, but a "how-to" manual) *all* diastolic murmurs should be considered pathologic. Diastolic murmurs can be caused by a patent arterial duct, leaking aortic or pulmonic valves, mitral or tricuspid stenosis, or relative mitral and tricuspid stenosis caused by increased blood flow across these two valves. But there is one common sound that is heard in diastole that is not pathologic, and that sound is a venous hum. The venous hum is probably related to

Table 2.2. Still's murmur	
Precordial activity	Normal
First heart sound (S1)	Normal
Second heart sound (S2)	Normal (splits with respiration)
Systolic murmur	
Grade	Grade 1–3
Location	Left sternal border, often widely throughout the precordium
Diastolic murmur	Venous hum
Femoral pulses	Normal

blood flow returning from the child's head and flowing from the superior vena cava to the right atrium. The venous hum is a continuous "whooshing" sound that sounds like listening to "a seashell at the seashore." This venous hum is commonly heard in children with Still's murmurs and is not pathologic. It is usually heard best with the child in the sitting position while the child is looking straightforward. Moving the child's head to either side often stops the venous hum (but not the Still's murmur). Venous hums are softer when the child is lying down and also are altered by light pressure to the right side of the neck, which temporarily stops blood flow through the right jugular venous system.

The second nuance with functional, innocent, and Still's murmurs is that the murmur changes with the position of the patient. Still's murmurs are loudest when the patient is supine and get softer when the patient stands. This is a very valuable physical examination finding, as the soft systolic vibratory murmur that disappears when the patient stands is very likely to be normal, and unlikely to be related to congenital heart disease. Remembering this physical exam trick is also important because the murmur in patients with hypertrophic cardiomyopathy, the most common cause of sudden death in young athletes, behaves just the opposite of a Still's murmur.

When any patient stands, gravity takes blood to the lower extremities, and therefore less blood is in the heart. With less blood filling the ventricle, the walls of the ventricles get closer together, and in the case of hypertrophic cardiomyopathy, the obstruction within the cavity of the left ventricle worsens (Fig. 2.2). Remember the very important distinction that a soft murmur associated with a normal first and second heart sound that gets softer when the patient's stand is very likely to be innocent murmur, but the soft systolic murmur that gets louder when the patient stands may be related to significant cardiac pathology.

The innocent murmur on the CD was recorded from an asymptomatic 4-year-old child with a loud vibratory systolic murmur. Please note that the first and second heart sounds are normal, and also note the very musical vibratory quality of this murmur. Click on the box marked standing, and a second recording obtained in the same patient shows how soft the murmur can get when the patient with a functional, innocent murmur stands (Table 2.3).

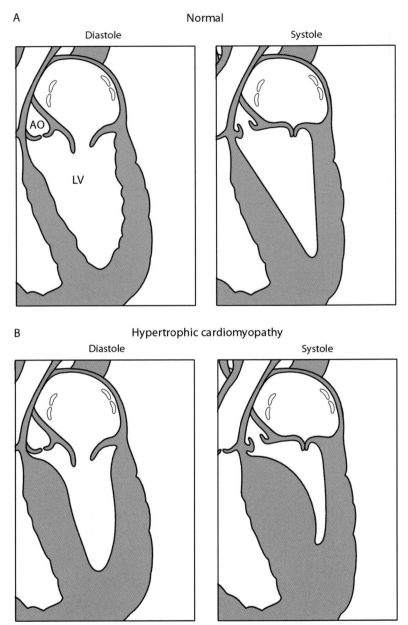

Fig. 2.2. Hypertrophic cardiomyopathy. Note the narrowing of the area between the left ventricle and the aorta that worsens with the patient standing

Table 2.3 What you hear on the CD-ROM

Functional murmur	Upper right sternal border	Upper left sternal border	Lower left sternal border	Apex
Supine				
First heart sound	Single, equal in intensity to S2	Single, equal in intensity to S2	Low pitched thud, shortly before the murmur begins	Soft single sound
Second heart sound	Single, equal in intensity to S1	Splits with respiration	Slightly louder than S1, splits with respiration, but not heard as well as it is at the upper left sternal border	Slightly louder than S1, splits with respiration, but not heard as well as it is at the upper left sternal border
Systole	Soft grade 1/6 ejection murmur	Soft grade 1/6 ejection murmur	Grade 2 to 3/6 vibratory musical murmur	Grade 2 to 3/6 vibratory musical murmur
Diastole	No murmur	No murmur	No murmur	No murmur
Standing				
First heart sound	Single, equal in intensity to S2	Single, equal in intensity to S2	Single, equal in intensity to S2	Single, equal in intensity to S2
Second heart sound	Single, equal in intensity to S1	Splits with respiration	Splits with respiration	Single, equal in intensity to S1
Systole	Soft grade 1/6 ejection murmur	Grade 1/6 musical vibratory murmur, softer than when the patient was lying down	Grade 1 to 2/6 musical vibratory murmur, softer than when the patient was lying down	Grade 1/6 musical vibratory murmur, softer than when the patient was lying down
Diastole	no murmur	no murmur	no murmur	no murmur

The Aortic Outflow Murmur

The third and final of the common innocent murmurs is the aortic outflow murmur of adolescents and young adults. The murmur is usually grade one or two in intensity, and is associated with normal first and second heart sounds. The murmur is heard best at the upper right sternal border (the aortic area) and is therefore felt to be secondary to blood flow in the left ventricular outflow tract. It is different from valvar aortic stenosis in that the patients do not have an ejection click. The murmur is often heard in athletes, who typically have a low resting heart rate and therefore a large stroke volume of blood flowing in the left ventricular outflow tract in systole. The outflow tract murmur of adolescents and young adults may also be confused with the murmur of hypertrophic cardiomyopathy. Standing a patient with hypertrophic cardiomyopathy should increase the murmur, whereas standing the patient with the aortic outflow murmur should result in either a decrease in the murmur, or no significant change.

It is important for the parents of a child with a functional or innocent murmur to know that their child is normal and that the child does not need restriction from any physical activity. In addition, the child does not need any special medical treatment. This is particularly confusing when the child goes to a dentist. Because patients with some cardiac pathology need to take antibiotics prior to certain dental procedures, the forms in dentist's office often ask simply "Do you have a heart murmur?". An affirmative answer to this question will often result in additional testing and anxiety. In the case of a child with a functional or innocent murmur, the proper

Table 2.4 Aortic outflow murmur	
Precordial activity	Normal
First heart sound (S1)	Normal
Second heart sound (S2)	Normal (splits with respiration)
Systolic murmur	
Grade	Grades 1–3
Location	Upper right sternal border
Diastolic murmur	None
Femoral pulses	Normal

answer to the question on the dental form is that the child *does not have a murmur*. This will eliminate anxiety and additional unnecessary testing (Table 2.4).

References

1. Danford DA (1995) Cost-effectiveness of echocardiography for evaluation of children with murmurs. Echocardiography 12:153–162

2. Shub C (2003) Echocardiography or auscultation? How to evaluate systolic murmurs. Can Family Physician 49:163–167

3. Pelech AN (2004) The physiology of cardiac auscultation. Pediatr Clin North Am 51(6):1515–1535

4. Gardiner HM (2002) Physiology of the developing human fetal heart. In: Anderson RH et al. (eds.) Paediatric cardiology Churchill Livingstone, London, pp 660–661

5. Walters M, Abelson HT (1996) Interpretation of the complete blood count. Pediatr Clin North Am 43(3):599–622

6. Rosenthal A (1984) How to distinguish between innocent and pathologic murmurs in childhood. Pediatr Clin of North Am 31:1229–1240

7. Still GH (1918) Common disorders and diseases of childhood, 3rd edn. Oxford University Press, London, p 495

Chapter 3
Atrial Septal Defects

M.E. McConnell, *Pediatric Heart Sounds*,
DOI: 10.1007/978-1-84628-684-1_3, © Springer-Verlag Lodon Limited 2008

Introduction

As discussed in Chapter 2, we all had an atrial septal defect at some point in our lives. Hopefully the defect that allowed oxygenated blood to flow from the right atrium to the left atrium while in the uterus closed after birth, but in approximately 0.075% of all children, the hole remains [1]. A tiny hole between the two atrial chambers does not cause excessive pulmonary blood flow and therefore cannot be diagnosed on physical examination. Rarely, a tiny hole in the atrial septum is important to diagnose, as some patients with small atrial septal defects may have passage of the deoxygenated blood from the right atrium to the left atrium or clots passing from the right atrium to the left atrium, causing a stroke. There is also some evidence suggesting that migraine headaches may improve after closure of a small patent foramen ovale [2]. But this is a murmur book, and the goal is to get the reader more comfortable using the stethoscope to diagnose innocent or pathologic murmurs. In my opinion, the ability to diagnose an atrial septal defect means that the listener is using his or her eyes, hands, ears, and brain to diagnose a subtle cardiac abnormality. For example, if a patient has a Grade 5 systolic murmur of aortic stenosis, it requires very little skill for the examiner to recognize that the patient has significant heart

Table 3.1. Comparison of the physical examination features of a patient with an atrial septal defect and a patient with a functional or innocent (normal) murmur

	Atrial septal defect	Innocent murmur
Precordial activity	Increased	Normal
First heart sound (S1)	Normal	Normal
Second heart sound (S2)	Widely split	Normal (splits with respiration)
Systolic murmur		
Grade	Grade 1–3	Grade 1–3
Location	Upper left sternal border	Left sternal border, often widely throughout the precordium
Quality	Crescendo decrescendo "flow"	Ejection crescendo decrescendo "musical"
Diastolic murmur	"Rumble" at the lower left sternal border	Venous hum
Femoral pulses	Normal	Normal

disease. The reported incidence of all congenital heart diseases varies between 0.5 and 1%, depending on the study. Patients with atrial septal defects are roughly 7–11% of all patients with congenital heart disease, meaning that roughly 1 in a 1,000 children will have a hemodynamically significant atrial septal defect [3]. Trying to tell the 1 in 1,000 patient with an atrial septal defect from the approximately 800 per 1,000 children who have a functional or innocent murmur requires a great deal of skill. Developing this skill is what this book and CD-ROM are all about. It would not be cost effective to refer all 800 children with murmurs to a pediatric cardiologist, but it certainly would not be optimal to miss the rare patient with an atrial septal defect (Table 3.1).

Anatomy

The atrial septum is a complex structure that contains a large hole in the center during fetal life (the foramen ovale, see Fig. 2.1). This hole allows oxygenated blood in the fetus to travel from the right atrium to the left atrium so it can go to perfuse the infant's brain. After birth, the foramen ovale should close, but in many people, a probe patent opening between the two atria remains. A persistent large

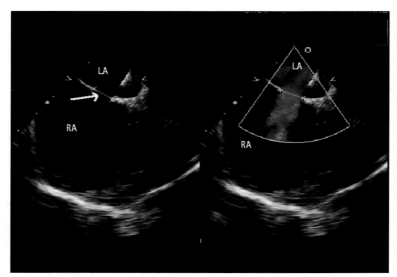

Fig. 3.1. *RA* right atrium, *LA* left atrium. The *arrow* points to the atrial septal defect. In the *frame on the right*, the *color* shows flow through the atrial defect

atrial defect may cause significant long-term health problems, such as recurrent pneumonia, failure to thrive, and eventually pulmonary hypertension (Fig. 3.1).

The life expectancy of a patient with a large atrial defect is significantly shortened, but if the defect is repaired before the development of pulmonary hypertension, the life expectancy of a patient with an atrial septal defect should be normal. As shown in the figure, the atrial septum may also have holes in locations other than the secundum septum, including the superior and inferior sinus venosus defects, the coronary sinus defects, and the ostium primum defects (Fig. 3.2). As this is an auscultation book, and not a pediatric cardiology text book, the discussion will center on the physical examination of a child and young adult with a hemodynamically significant atrial septal defect.

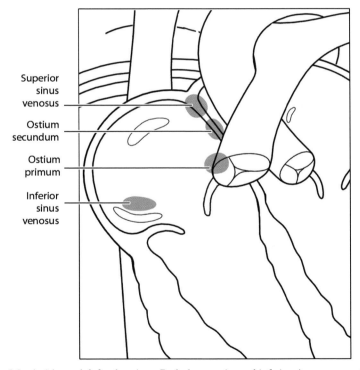

Fig. 3.2. Atrial septal defect locations. Both the superior and inferior sinus venosus ASDs may be associated with right to left shunting, even in the absence of pulmonary hypertension. The secundum defect is the most common, and is in the location of the fetal foramen ovale

Inspection

Inspection of the older child with a hemodynamically significant atrial septal defect may show "chest asymmetry." When looking from the head to the feet, the anterior chest wall bulges on the left side because the heart beneath the left chest is enlarged (see Fig. 3.3).

Palpation

The cardiac output in a child is normally about $5\,L/(min*m)^2$ body surface area. This means that for each minute in a child of about 7 years age, the heart pumps 5 L of blood from each ventricle (or 10 L/min total). In a patient with a large atrial septal defect, the heart may pump three or four times as much blood to the lungs as it pumps to the aorta. This means that instead of the heart pumping a total of 10 l/min, it now pumps 25 l/min! Palpation on the left chest in a patient with this increased cardiac output will reveal a left parasternal lift, meaning the overactive ventricle is pushing against the chest wall with systole. The only way to differentiate this abnormal physical finding from the precordial activity of a normal person is to get into the habit of precordial palpation on all patients you examine. When the rare patient comes along with increased precordial activity due to increased cardiac output, the difference in precordial activity between that patient and a normal will hopefully be obvious.

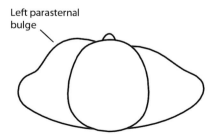

Left parasternal bulge

Fig. 3.3. Left parasternal bulge caused by asymmetrical chest wall growth. The enlarged right ventricle causes the left side of the chest wall to deform anteriorly in comparison to the right chest wall

Auscultation

After inspecting the chest and palpating for a parasternal lift, use the stethoscope diaphragm at the lower left sternal border and listen carefully for the first heart sound. In a patient with an atrial septal defect, the closure of the mitral and tricuspid valves should be easily heard. The first sound should be single or narrowly split, and there are no clicks. Now use the diaphragm and listen at the upper left sternal border for the second heart sound. In Chapter 1, we learned that the second heart sound is caused by the closure of the pulmonic and aortic valves and that the pulmonary components of the second heart sound "splits" and moves away from the aortic closure sound when the patient takes a deep breath. This is because the deep breath brings additional venous return to the right side of the heart, and the right ventricle takes longer to eject its contents. The pulmonary valve therefore closes after the aortic valve. In a patient with an atrial septal defect, the blood flow flowing from the left atrium to the right atrium through the atrial defect meets with the superior vena cava blood and the inferior vena cava blood and then flows into the right ventricle. Therefore, the right ventricle always has more blood in it than the left ventricle, and the pulmonary valve closure sound always resembles the second heart sound heard when a patient takes a deep breath. This means the pulmonic component closes after the aortic component. This is also known as a "fixed split" second heart sound. It sounds like thump (the first heart sound) then thump thump. Another cause of a fixed split second heart sound is a complete right bundle branch block. This may be post surgical or idiopathic. In complete right bundle branch block, the right ventricle always depolarizes after the left ventricle and the pulmonary valve always closes after the aortic valve (Fig. 3.4). In summary, in a patient with atrial septal defect, the precordial activity is increased, the first heart sound is normal, and the second heart sound is widely split.

Now we get to the murmur in patients with atrial septal defects. One of the big problems with diagnosing ASDs and why auscultation is so important to perform properly is that there are many people with large atrial septal defects who have *no systolic murmur*! Therefore, the presence or absence of a systolic murmur is not necessarily the reason a patient should be referred to a pediatric cardiologist. You may have no murmur and have

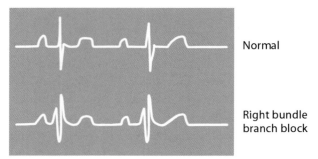

Normal

Right bundle
branch block

Fig. 3.4. Complete right bundle branch block recorded in V1 in comparison to a normal EKG. The wide QRS complex means that the electrical impulse moves slowly through the myocardium, and the right ventricle depolarizes after the left, causing the right ventricle to eject its contents after the left ventricle. The pulmonary valve therefore closes after the aortic valve, giving a "fixed split"

significant congenital heart disease or have a murmur and have no congenital heart disease. In a patient with an atrial septal defect, the murmur (if they have one) is caused by blood flow from the right ventricle into the lungs. Because of the extra blood flow, the pulmonary outflow tract may dilate over time. This extra blood flow may go from the right ventricle to the lungs without making noise (and therefore the patient will have no systolic murmur). The systolic murmur at the upper left sternal border caused by the extra flow into the lungs starts after S1 and is therefore an ejection "diamond-shaped" murmur. The murmur is grade 3 or less and may radiate to the lungs. The murmur does not change with position. Because the murmur is soft, not necessarily harsh, and does not obscure the first heart sound, it is often confused with a functional or innocent murmur.

Another physical exam finding that separates patients with atrial septal defects from patients with functional or innocent murmurs is the presence of a "diastolic rumble." This sound, which is well heard on the CD-ROM, is caused by the extra blood flow across the tricuspid valve in diastole. Because it is a very low-pitch sound, a diastolic rumble is heard best with the bell of the stethoscope placed at the lower left sternal border (the tricuspid area). Press down with the bell, and it will act like a diaphragm, and the higher pitched sounds, like S1, S2, and possibly the pulmonary flow murmur, will be easily audible. Now let up on the bell, and it will begin to transmit the lower frequency sounds. One of these low-frequency sounds is a

Table 3.2. What you hear on the CD-ROM

Atrial septal defect	Upper right sternal border	Upper left sternal border	Lower left sternal border	Apex
First heart sound	Not audible	Single, slightly softer than S2	Low-pitched thud, slightly softer than S2	Soft single sound
Second heart sound	Single	Widely split, does not vary with respiration	Slightly louder than S1, single	Single sound, slightly louder than S1
Systole	Grade 1 to 2/6 ejection murmur	Grade 2 to 3/6 systolic ejection murmur	Grade 1 to 2/6 ejection murmur	Grade 1/6 ejection murmur
Diastole	No murmur	No murmur	Grade 1 to 2/4 low-pitched rumble, an "absence of silence"	Very faint, grade 1/4 diastolic rumble

diastolic rumble of a patient with an atrial septal defect. Because there is no significant pressure gradient from the right atrium to the right ventricle in diastole, the soft diastolic flow rumble may be very difficult to hear. This sound is like "Niagara Falls from miles away," a soft rumbling sound. It is also described as "an absence of silence" (see CD-ROM waveform comparison, Table 3.2).

The CD-ROM recording is best appreciated using good computer speakers, including a subwoofer, or good headphones. Listen at the lower left sternal border, and concentrate on diastole. After several cardiac cycles, it should become obvious that after the second heart sound, the heart does not become silent because there is a soft diastolic rumbling sound. If you still cannot appreciate this subtle auscultatory finding, go to the normal heart sounds and listen at the lower left sternal border. Note the silence in diastole. Now return to the ASD portion of the CD-ROM and compare the diastolic sounds. The lack of "silence" after the second heart sound in the patient with an atrial septal defect will hopefully be evident.

I realize that there is not enough time in the day to do a complete, extensive cardiac physical examination on every patient who comes to a busy pediatric or family practice office. Before considering referral to a pediatric cardiologist for evaluation of a murmur, I would strongly encourage you to go through the complete exam as outlined above and ask yourself, "Does this patient have an atrial septal defect?". This should remind you to look for a left parasternal bulge and then to feel the precordial activity, feeling for increased cardiac activity. It will also remind you to listen critically for the first and second heart sounds and to listen throughout the precordium in systole and in diastole with both the bell and the diaphragm. Have the patient stand and note if the murmur gets softer. Hopefully by following this routine, you will refer fewer patients with functional or innocent murmurs and appropriately refer patients who might have an atrial septal defect.

It is also important to note that although all children who have large hemodynamically atrial septal defects are born with a defect in the atrial septum, the hole may grow over time. Therefore, their physical examination may change over time as the right ventricle dilates and the amount of pulmonary blood flow increases. It is unlikely for a baby to have a classic atrial septal defect exam because it takes time for the right ventricle to dilate enough so that the RV volume is significantly greater than the LV volume. Until the RV volume significantly exceeds the LV volume, the precordial activity will remain normal, and the second heart sound will remain normal as well. The patient also will not have a diastolic rumble. The point is that the physical examination is dynamic and will hopefully become more obvious over time. If you see an asymptomatic child and you are not certain if the child has a functional murmur or an atrial septal defect, re-evaluation in the next year may suggest the correct diagnosis. There is no urgent reason to know whether an asymptomatic child has an atrial septal defect or a functional murmur, as patients with atrial septal defects do not require antibiotic prophylaxis, and when the patient is asymptomatic, closure of the defect is elective.

Subacute Bacterial Endocarditis Prophylaxis Recommendations (SBE)

According to the guidelines published by the American Heart Association in 2007, patients with atrial septal defects do not require antibiotic prophylaxis at times of endocarditis risk [4].

References

1. Samanek M, Slavik Z, Zborilova B, Hrobonova V, Voriskova M, Skovranek J (1989) Prevalence, treatment, and outcome of heart disease in live-born children: a prospective analysis of 91,823 live-born children. Pediatr Cardiol 10(4):205–211

2. Post MC, Thijs V, Herroelen L, Budts WI (2007) Closure of a patent foramen ovale is associated with a decrease in prevalence of migraine. Neurology 62(8):1439–1440

3. Beerman LB, Zuberbuhler JR (2002) Arial septal defect. In: Anderson RH et al (eds.) Paediatric cardiology.. Churchill Livingstone, London, pp 901–930

4. Wilson W, Taubert K, Gewitz M et al. (2007) Prevention of infective endocarditis. Guidelines from the American Heart Association. Rheumatic Fever, Endocarditis, and Kawasaki Disease Committee, Council on Cardiovascular Disease in the Young, and the Council on Clinical Cardiology, Council on Cardiovascular Surgery and Anesthesia, and the Quality of Care and Outcomes Research Interdisciplinary Working Group 2007. Circulation April 19

Chapter 4
Ventricular Septal Defects

M.E. McConnell, *Pediatric Heart Sounds*,
DOI: 10.1007/978-1-84628-684-1_4, © Springer-Verlag London Limited 2008

Incidence

Defects in the interventricular septum are common. A recent study suggested that the incidence was as high as 2–4% of all newborn infants [1, 2] Understanding when these defects might present clinically is important in understanding the physiology of the disorder. When infants are born, until the arterial duct and the atrial septal defect close, the pressures in the right and left ventricles may be similar. As the pulmonary vascular resistance drops, and the arterial duct closes, the right and left ventricles will have different pressures. This drop in pulmonary vascular resistance, and therefore right ventricular pressure, is usually complete by 6 weeks of age. The ability to hear a murmur of a ventricular septal defect depends on the difference in pressure from the left to the right ventricle. If, for example, the pulmonary vascular resistance drops quickly, the harsh murmur of a restrictive ventricular septal may be heard in the first few days of life. On the other hand, if the pulmonary vascular resistance is high, then the pressure in the right ventricle will remain high, and there will be little pressure difference between the LV and the RV. In this case, it may be very difficult to hear the murmur of a ventricular septal defect.

Anatomy

Ventricular septal defects are named based on their location within the ventricular septum. The right ventricle wraps around the conical left ventricle (Fig. 4.1) One way to visualize this relationship is to use your right hand, with the palm pointing toward your chest, and the hand slightly cupped. The thumb of your right hand would be in the tricuspid valve, and the fingers of the right hand would be in the right ventricular outflow tract. All along this three-dimensional structure, a defect could join the right ventricle with the left. If the defect was in the posterior part of the RV, near the tricuspid valve (the thumb), it would be called an inlet ventricular septal defect. These defects are usually associated with abnormalities of the tricuspid and mitral valves, and are not likely to close spontaneously. These inlet ventricular septal defects are common in children with Down syndrome. When the inlet ventricular septal defect is also associated with an inferior atrial septal defect (a so-called ostium

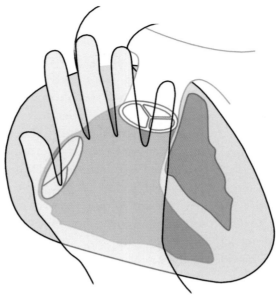

Fig. 4.1. The normal relationship between the right and the left ventricle. The right ventricle wraps around the conical left ventricle. See text

primum ASD) they are called atrioventricular septal defects or atrioventricular canal defects.

Defects near the aortic valve on the left side, and the tricuspid valve on the right side are called membranous or perimembranous ventricular septal defects (Fig. 4.2). Ventricular septal defects vary in size, and may close spontaneously. Often they are large enough and have a large enough volume of blood flowing through the defect that the children cannot eat and grow well, and surgical intervention is warranted. These perimembranous defects would be near the junction of the thumb and the palm, when using the example above (see Fig. 4.1).

Ventricular septal defects in the palm of the hand, potentially going into the apex of both ventricles are called muscular ventricular septal defects. These defects are often small, but may be multiple (the so-called "Swiss-cheese" septum). Small muscular defects are common in normal newborns, and have a tendency to close very quickly. One study suggests that about 75% of muscular defects close within the first year of life [2].

The last location of ventricular septal defects is in the outlet septum. If the defect is beneath the right aortic cusp and the

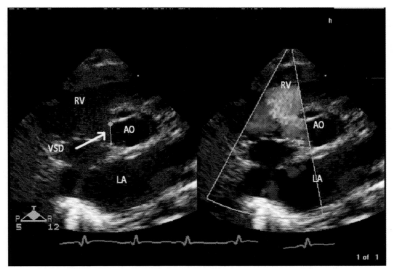

Fig. 4.2. A perimembranous ventricular septal defect shown in the short axis view. *LA* left atrium, *RV* right ventricle, *AO* aorta. The *arrow* shows the large ventricular septal defect (VSD). The *right side panel* shows blood flow through the defect

pulmonary valve it is called a subarterial or a doubly committed ventricular septal defect. This would be in the region of the fingers in the hand example. Defects in this location are less likely than muscular defects to close spontaneously, and are more likely to be associated with intracardiac problems like aortic valve insufficiency (see Fig. 4.1). The aortic insufficiency may be seen in as many as 65% of patients with subarterial ventricular septal defects [3]. Some studies suggest that the aortic valve abnormality that may occur with a subarterial ventricular septal defect might be prevented by early closure of the ventricular septal defect [4].

Physiology

The physiology of a ventricular septal defect depends on the amount of blood flowing through the defect, and associated abnormalities, such as a patent arterial duct or mitral valve regurgitation. In a patient with an isolated ventricular septal defect, the amount of blood flowing through the defect depends on the size of the hole and the pulmonary vascular resistance, as discussed above (see CD-ROM about VSD). If the pulmonary vascular resistance is low, and the hole is moderate in size, there might be a great deal of blood flowing from the left ventricle through the ventricular septal defect, and into the right ventricle. This blood will subsequently flow from the right ventricle into the pulmonary artery. Patients with a large left-to-right shunt often have increased work of breathing, because their lungs are overfilled with blood. The increased cardiac output causes an increased metabolic rate, and the increased work of breathing often means that the infants with large left-to-right shunts cannot eat as well as a child who breathes normally. The total energy expenditure in infants with ventricular septal defects and congestive heart failure symptoms can be 50% higher than the energy expenditure of age matched control infants [5]. The amount of blood flow through the defect is also a variable phenomenon, and it can increase as the pulmonary vascular resistance decreases. It is important to note that the left-to-right shunt of a ventricular septal defect sends oxygenated blood from the left ventricle back into the right ventricle. The patients are therefore not cyanotic (blue) unless there is pulmonary hypertension. In patients with large ventricular septal defects, there may not be a pressure difference between the left and the right ventricle and there may not be a classic ventricular septal defect murmur. There are rare children with large ventricular septal defects who never drop their pulmonary vascular resistance, and therefore who never have signs of a large left-to-right shunt. These patients can be very difficult to diagnose, unless the observer does a careful cardiac examination. Children with Down syndrome have a 50% incidence of significant congenital heart disease. Rarely, a child with Down syndrome will have high pulmonary vascular resistance at birth, and therefore will not have a large left-to-right shunt. They may remain asymptomatic for many years, until the pulmonary vasculature becomes so damaged that the patient begins to shunt blue blood from the right ventricle to the left side of the circulation. This condition is known as Eisenmengers syndrome (see CD-ROM large VSD with pulmonary hypertension). At this point, the children are not operable, as an operation to close either the atrial or ventricular defect is likely to cause worsening symptoms or death.One way to avoid this scenario is to refer all children with Down syndrome for at least one cardiac evaluation. Because the incidence of disease is so high (50% compared to a general population of less than 1%)the chances of finding an abnormality are very high.

Natural History

The natural history of a patient with a ventricular septal defect is quite variable. Many of the small defects close spontaneously, especially the muscular ventricular septal defects. One study showed that muscular ventricular septal defects had a 69% chance of spontaneous closure within the first 6 years of life. This same study showed that muscular ventricular septal defects were also unlikely to require surgical intervention, with only 1 in 39 patients requiring surgery [2].Perimembranous ventricular septal defects have a higher likelihood of causing significant symptoms, and therefore are more likely to require surgical intervention. Spontaneous closure occurred in 28% of patients with a perimembranous ventricular septal defect followed for 6 years, but surgical intervention to close the defect was needed in 41% over the same time period. Even if a membranous ventricular septal defect is felt to be "asymptomatic" and not large enough to warrant surgical intervention, long-term complications are common. The incidence of endocarditis is estimated at 14.5/10,000 patient years [6]. Other complications of even small ventricular septal defects include subaortic obstruction, aortic valve insufficiency, muscular right ventricular outflow tract obstruction, and congestive heart failure. Aortic valve insufficiency can be seen in up to 7.5% of adults with perimembranous or subarterial ventricular septal defects, and is often progressive [7]. A recent study suggested that the 8-year event-free survival for adults with small ventricular septal defects was over 95% [8]. Events in their study were defined as death, endocarditis, or need for surgical closure of the ventricular septal defect. Other authors suggest that the risk of the above-listed complications in adults with small ventricular septal defects is as high as 25% [9].

Medical Management

Because most ventricular septal defects close spontaneously, or at least get smaller over time, if the child is able to eat reasonably well and grow, surgery should be avoided. In some infants, the large left-to-right shunt through the ventricular septal defect causes increased pulmonary circulation, resulting in increased work of breathing. This is coupled with decreased systemic blood flow, as the blood leaving the left ventricle can more easily flow through the VSD and into the pulmonary circulation than flow through the aortic valve and into the systemic circulation. Decreased systemic blood flow results in the activation of the renin–angiotensin–aldosterone system and the sympathetic nervous system. The infants are often irritable, feed poorly, are pale, and have increased work of breathing [10]. Traditionally these infants are treated with digoxin and diuretics, although the evidence that these medications are effective for this hemodynamic derangement is lacking [11]. In adult patients with congestive heart failure, treatment with medications to block the elevated neurohormones, such as angiotensin converting enzyme inhibitors and beta blockers have been shown to improve survival significantly. Although the mechanism of congestive heart failure in infants with ventricular septal defects is very different from the mechanism in most adults with congestive heart failure, the neurohormonal elevation is similar, suggesting that possibly the medications that are effective for adults with congestive heart failure might be useful for symptomatic patients with large left-to-right shunts [12, 13].

Surgical Options

If the infant is not thriving, surgical closure of the ventricular septal defect may be the safest course. In most major centers, closure of a membranous ventricular septal defect, even in a small child, carries a mortality rate of less than 1%. Because chronic congestive heart failure is not benign, with infants at risk for RSV infections and possibly neurologic abnormalities, early intervention to close ventricular septal defects in symptomatic infants should be considered [14].

For some patients, closure of the ventricular septal defect surgically carries increased risk. This might include patients with large muscular ventricular septal defects that are not easily closed surgically. For some of these patients, closure of the defect in the catheterization laboratory may be the safest procedure. In 2004, Knauth published a 13-year experience involving 170 patients with ventricular septal defects "selected for device closure if they had 1 or more VSDs that were ascertained to result in sufficient hemodynamic derangement to warrant intervention and either a type of VSD that was technically difficult to close surgically or an overall medical condition with associated surgical risks sufficient to justify the known and potential unknown risks of the device." A total of 69% of the patients had muscular ventricular septal defects, and the remainder had either intentionally fenestrated VSD patches or postoperative residual defects along the margin of patches used to close VSDs in the membranous or outflow portions of the septum. A total of 296 devices were implanted in the 170 patients. There were 332 adverse events reported in 153 of the 170 patients (90%), including hemorrhage, arrhythmia, new onset regurgitation of the aortic or tricuspid valve, death, and need for device explantation. The authors felt that only one patient died as a result of the device implantation, and that the majority had a significant decrease in the size of the shunt through the ventricular septal defect. As new devices become available, catheter closure of ventricular septal defects may become the preferred method [15].

Physical Examination

The physical examination in a patient with a ventricular septal defect varies greatly depending on the size of the defect, the pulmonary vascular resistance, and the amount of blood flowing through the defect.

Small Muscular Ventricular Septal Defects

The tiny muscular ventricular septal defects discussed earlier allow very little blood to flow from the left to the right ventricle, and are also associated with normal pulmonary vascular resistance. Patients with small muscular ventricular septal defects would have normal precordial activity, because the heart is pumping a normal amount of blood. It would also be unusual to palpate a thrill in a patient with a small muscular ventricular septal defect. The shunt through the ventricular septum starts as the AV valves are closing (the "isovolumic contraction phase") and the murmur therefore "obscures" the first heart sound. The murmur is harsh, not musical like a functional or innocent murmur. In many small muscular ventricular septal

Table 4.1. Small muscular VSD

Precordial activity	Normal
First heart sound (S1)	Obscured
Second heart sound (S2)	Normal (splits with respiration)
Systolic murmur	
Grade	Grade 1–3
Location	lower left sternal border, may stop in mid-systole
Diastolic murmur	None
Femoral pulses	Normal

defect patients, the murmur stops before the second heart sound. This is because the muscular ventricular septal defect is so small that it actually closes during systole, cutting off the blood flow from the left to the right ventricle. In patients with a small muscular ventricular septal defect, the pulmonary artery pressure should be normal, and therefore the second heart sound should split and move normally with respiration. The pulses will be normal (Table 4.1).

Moderate Ventricular Septal Defects

In patients with moderate ventricular septal defects, the physical examination again depends a great deal on the size of the defect, the pulmonary vascular resistance, and the amount of flow through the defect. The location of the moderate defects is not critical to the physical examination, but rarely there can be differentiating factors that point to the location of the defect within the interventricular septum.

Inspection of the chest might show a left parasternal bulge, caused by chest deformation secondary to the large heart (see Fig. 3.3). Also on inspection the child who is in significant congestive heart failure might have "Harrison's Groove", a longitudinal depression at the site of the insertion of the diaphragm. If the patient has a large left-to-right shunt through the ventricular septal defect, there might be three or four times as much blood flowing into the pulmonary artery as is flowing into the aorta. The heart may then be pumping two or three times as much blood as a normal child, and this difference should be easily palpable by placing your hand on the precordium. Often a parasternal thrill is palpable, caused by the rapid flow of blood from the left ventricle into the right ventricle, and the subsequent vibration on the anterior chest wall. The first heart sound will be obscured by the rapid flow of blood from the left to the right ventricle, and the harsh systolic murmur is often best heard at the left lower sternal border. If the murmur is higher on the left sternal border, it may be the murmur of a subarterial ventricular septal defect or possibly severe pulmonary outflow tract obstruction. Occasionally, the tricuspid valve tissue that partially closes the perimembranous ventricular septal defects can "pop" during systole, causing an early systolic ejection sound. The second heart will depend on the pulmonary artery pressure. If the pulmonary artery pressure is normal, the second heart sound is normal, splitting and moving with respiration. If the pulmonary artery pressure is elevated, the second heart sound can be loud and single. Because a large extra amount of blood flows through the mitral valve in diastole, a low-pitched "diastolic rumble" is often audible in children with moderate ventricular septal defects and large left-to-right shunts. This low-pitched diastolic sound is analogous to the diastolic rumble audible in patients with hemodynamically significant atrial septal defects, except that in ASD patients the rumble is across the tricuspid valve and in VSD patients the rumble is across the mitral valve. The rumble is best appreciated using the bell of the stethoscope placed at the apex (the mitral area). Press down with the bell and it will act like a diaphragm, enhancing the high-frequency noises. Now, lessen the pressure, and the bell will transmit more low-frequency sounds. The rumble sounds like a distant noise after S2, when the heart should be quiet (see CD-ROM waveforms). Audible flow across the mitral valve will indicate that the pulmonary to systemic blood flow ratio will be at least 2 to 1 [16].

The ventricular septal defect recording on the CD-ROM is an S1 coincident, harsh holosystolic murmur that is loudest at the lower left sternal border. The second heart sound splits and moves with respiration, implying that the pulmonary artery pressure is normal. This also implies that the defect is relatively small, since there can be a pressure difference between the two ventricles. In the recording, there is no diastolic rumble audible at the apex, implying that the left-to-right shunt does not exceed 2 to 1. In this recording, because the infant was very active and the recording was

Table 4.2. Moderate ventricular septal defect

Precordial activity	Possibly increased, possible thrill
First heart sound (S1)	Obscured
Second heart sound (S2)	Normal (splits with respiration)
Systolic murmur	
Grade	Grade 3–6
Location	lower left sternal border
Diastolic murmur	Possible "rumble" heard at the mitral area
Femoral pulses	Normal

"noisy", there are only two cardiac cycles "looped". What this means is, if you are having trouble hearing the second heart sound split, this is a good recording to practice this skill. There is a cardiac cycle with an S1 coincident holosystolic murmur, followed by a single second heart sound. The second cardiac cycle has a holosystolic murmur, followed by a split second heart sound. If you get the rhythm, you should eventually be able to hear the difference between the single second heart sound and the split second heart sound (Table 4.2).

Large Ventricular Septal Defects

Patients with large ventricular septal defects will have widely different physical examinations depending on their pulmonary artery pressure and pulmonary blood flow. If the defect is large and the pulmonary vascular resistance is low, the patients will have a large left-to-right shunt. Their physical examination will be as described for the moderate ventricular septal defect above with some notable exceptions. There may be a left parasternal bulge and Harrison's groove, depending on the age of the child. The precordial activity will be increased because there will be a great deal of extra cardiac output. Because the large ventricular septal defect allows the pressures in the right and left ventricle to equalize, there is not a classic "holosystolic" murmur that would ordinarily obscure the first heart sound. Therefore the first heart sound in a patient with a large unrestrictive ventricular septal defect is normal, audible at the lower left sternal border. The excessive pulmonary blood flow

Table 4.3. Large ventricular septal defect with large left-to-right shunt

Precordial activity	Increased
First heart sound (S1)	May be audible
Second heart sound (S2)	Narrowly split
Systolic murmur	
Grade	Grade 3–6
Location	Upper left sternal border
Diastolic murmur	Possible "rumble" heard at the mitral area
Femoral pulses	Normal

causes the systolic murmur, and this murmur is heard best at the upper left sternal border, in the pulmonary area.If the diastolic pressure in the pulmonary artery is low, the second heart sound might split, but if the diastolic pressure is high, the second heart sound can be single and loud. If the left-to-right shunt exceeds 2 to 1, there should be a diastolic rumble audible over the mitral area (Table 4.3).

The final variation on the ventricular septal defect theme is the patient with Eisenmenger's syndrome. Dr. Eisenmenger described a patient in 1879 who had cyanosis and was later found at autopsy to have a ventricular septal defect and aortic overriding. This means that the aorta partially arose from the right ventricle and partially arose from the left ventricle. Many years after the initial description, Eisenmenger's syndrome came to refer a patient with a left-to-right shunt (VSD, ASD, or PDA) who developed pulmonary vascular disease, and then began to shunt right to left, leading to cyanosis. This is different from Eisenmenger's original hypothesis, in that he thought the presence of the aorta partially above the right ventricle would lead to cyanosis [17]. We now know that even if the aorta arises partially from the right ventricle, unless there is obstruction to pulmonary blood flow either from pulmonary stenosis (like in tetralogy of Fallot) or pulmonary hypertension (like in what is now known as Eisenmeinger's syndrome) the patient will not have cyanosis (see VSD with pulmonary hypertension figure on the CD-ROM).

Patients with large ventricular septal defects and pulmonary hypertension may have a palpable right ventricular impulse, but often have no unusual precordial activity. Since the defect is large

Table 4.4. Large ventricular septal defect with pulmonary hypertension

Precordial activity	May be normal
First heart sound (S1)	May be audible
Second heart sound (S2)	Single and loud
Systolic murmur	
Grade	May have no murmur
Location	–
Diastolic murmur	Possibly a pulmonary valve insufficiency murmur
Femoral pulses	Normal

and there is no obstruction between the two ventricles, the first heart sound is audible and normal. The pulmonary vascular disease prevents the heart from pumping an excessive amount of blood to the lungs and therefore there is no systolic murmur, either through the ventricular septal defect or across the pulmonary outflow tract. The second heart sound is loud and single, as the pressure pushing the pulmonary valve closed is the same pressure pushing the aortic valve closed. Diastolic murmurs caused by a leaking pulmonary valve are common in patients with Eisenmenger's syndrome (Tables 4.4, 4.5).

Table 4.5. What you hear on the CD-ROM

Ventricular septal defect	Upper right sternal border	Upper left sternal border	Lower left sternal border	Apex
First heart sound	Not audible	Not audible	Not audible	Not audible
Second heart sound	Single	Splits with every other breath, because of the editing of the sound file	Faint and splits every other beat	Faint and splits every other beat
Systole	Grade 2 to 3/6 harsh murmur	Grade 2/6 harsh murmur	Grade 3/6 harsh	Grade 2 to 3/6 harsh murmur
Diastole	No murmur	No murmur	No murmur	No murmur

Subacute Bacterial Endocarditis Prophylaxis Recommendations (SBE)

According to the guidelines published by the American Heart Association in 2007, patients with ventricular septal defects do not require antibiotic prophylaxis at times of endocarditis risk, unless they have had a prior case of endocarditis. Rarely, some postoperative patients who have residual ventricular septal defects will need SBE prophylaxis [18].

Summary

Patients with ventricular septal defects are common. The physical examination can vary in many different ways, depending on the size of the defect and the amount of blood flowing through the defect. In a patient with a moderate-sized ventricular septal defect, there may be a palpable thrill, increased precordial activity, an obscured first heart sound, a normal second heart sound, and a harsh systolic murmur at the mid-left sternal border.

References

1. Sands A, Lynch C, Casey F, Craig B, Dornan J, Mulholland C (1998). Ventricular septal defects: the relationship of social class and area of residence to occurrence rate Fetal Diagn Ther 13(Suppl I):148

2. Hiraishi S, Agata Y, Nowatari M et al. (1992) Incidence and natural course of trabecular ventricular septal defect: two dimensional echocardiography and color Doppler flow imaging study.J Pediatr 120:409–415.

3. Komai H. Naito Y. Fujiwara K. Noguchi Y. Nishimura Y. Uemura S (1997) Surgical strategy for doubly committed subarterial ventricular septal defect with aortic cusp prolapse. Ann Thoracic Surg 64(4):1146–1149

4. Kobayashi J, Koike K, Senzaki H, Kobayashi T, Tsunemoto M, Ishizawa A, Ohta Y, Shimada M, Omoto R (1999) Correlation of anatomic and hemodynamic features with aortic valve leaflet deformity in doubly committed subarterial ventricular septal defect. Heart Vessels 14(5):240-245

5. Farrell AG, Schamberger MS, Olson IL, Leitch CA (2001) Large left-to-right shunts and congestive heart failure increase total energy expenditure in infants with ventricular septal defect. Am J Cardiol 87(9):1128–1131, A10

6. Gersony WM, Hayes CJ, Driscoll DJ, et al. (1993) Bacterial endocarditis in patients with aortic stenosis, pulmonary stenosis or ventricular septal defects. Circulation 87(Suppl I):1121–1126

7. Eroglu AG, Oztunc F, Saltik L, Dedeoglu S, Bakari S, Ahunbay G (2003) Aortic valve prolapse and aortic regurgitation in patients with ventricular septal defect. Pediatr Cardiol 24(1):36–39

8. Gabriel HM, Heger M, Innerhofer P, Zehetgruber M, Mundigler G, Wimmer M, Maurer G, Baumgartner H (2002) Long-term outcome of patients with ventricular septal defect considered not to require surgical closure during childhood. J Am College Cardiol 39(6):1066–1071

9. Neumayer U, Stone S, Somerville J (1998) Small ventricular septal defects in adults. Eur Heart J 19(10):1573–1582

10. Kay JD, Colan SD, Graham TP Jr (2001) Congestive heart failure in pediatric patients. AHJ 142(5)

11. Kimball TR, Daniels SR, Meyer RA, Hannon DW, Tian J, Shukla R, Schwartz DC (1991) Effect of digoxin on contractility and symptoms in infants with a large ventricular septal defect. Am J Cardiol 68(13):1377–1382

12. Ross RD, Daniels SR, Schwartz DC, Hannon DW, Kaplan S (1987) Return of plasma norepinephrine to normal after

resolution of congestive heart failure in congenital heart disease. Am J Cardiol 60(16):1411–1413

13. Buchhorn R, Hulpke-Wette M, Ruschewski W, Ross RD, Fielitz J, Pregla R, Hetzer R, Regitz-Zagrosek V (2003) Effects of therapeutic beta blockade on myocardial function and cardiac remodelling in congenital cardiac disease. Cardiol Young 13(1):36–43

14. Limperopoulos C, Majnemer A, Shevell MI, et al. (2000) Neurodevelopmental status of newborns and infants with congenital heart defects before and after open heart surgery. J Pediatr 137:638–645

15. Knauth AL, Lock JE, Perry SB, McElhinney DB, Gauvreau K, Landzberg MJ, Rome JJ, Hellenbrand WE, Ruiz CE, Jenkins KJ (2004) Transcatheter device closure of congenital and postoperative residual ventricular septal defects. Circulation 110(5):501–507

16. Tynan M, Anderson RH (2002) Ventricular septal defect. In:Anderson RH et al. (eds.) Paediatric cardiology. Churchill Livingstone, London, pp 983–1014

17. Wilkinson JL (2000). In: Moller JH and Hoffman JIE (eds.) Ventricular septal defect in pediatric cardiovascular medicine. Churchill Livingstone, New York, pp 289–309

18. Wilson W, Taubert K, Gewitz M et al. (2007) Prevention of infective endocarditis. Guidelines from the American Heart Association. A Guideline From the American Heart Association Rheumatic Fever, Endocarditis, and Kawasaki Disease Committee, Council on Cardiovascular Disease in the Young, and the Council on Clinical Cardiology, Council on Cardiovascular Surgery and Anesthesia, and the Quality of Care and Outcomes Research Interdisciplinary Working Group 2007. Circulation April 19

Chapter 5
Patent Arterial Duct

M.E. McConnell, *Pediatric Heart Sounds*,
DOI: 10.1007/978-1-84628-684-1_5, © Springer-Verlag London Limited 2008

Introduction

The arterial duct, also known as a patent ductus arteriosus (PDA) is a relatively uncommon congenital malformation. Although all newborns have a patent arterial duct, it should close shortly after birth. Because the duct closes spontaneously in the vast majority of infants, persistence into later life is relatively rare. The estimated incidence of a PDA in children by 4 years of age is about 3/10,000 children.

Anatomy

The arterial duct is an intrauterine structure that connects the aorta and the pulmonary artery. In utero, the ductus carries relatively deoxygenated blood from the fetal right ventricle into the descending aorta, so that the deoxygenated blood perfuses the placenta. There the blood is oxygenated and returns to the fetal heart, coursing through the umbilical vein through the venous duct and into the right atrium (see Fig. 2.1). After birth, many biochemical signals, including the increase in oxygen level in the newborn circulation, act on the ductus to cause closure. The ductus is encircled with muscular tissue that constricts, so that within the first 24 h of post-natal life, the ductus is functionally closed in most newborns. If these signals do not cause the ductus to close, the patient will have a patent arterial duct, or PDA (Fig. 5.1).

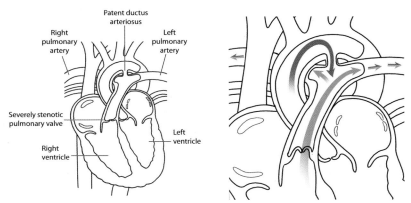

Fig. 5.1. The patent arterial duct. Note the connection between the aorta and the pulmonary artery, allowing the oxygenated (red) blood to flow from the aorta into the pulmonary artery

Physiology

While the fetus is in the uterus, the arterial duct is necessary to allow blood to leave the right ventricle, flow into the main pulmonary artery, and then down into the aorta. After the infant is born, the pulmonary artery pressure drops significantly, and therefore the aortic pressure is higher than the pulmonary artery pressure. If the duct remains patent, the aortic high-pressure blood will flow into the low-pressure pulmonary artery in both systole and diastole. The amount of this blood flow depends on the size of the ductus, as well as the difference in pressure and vascular resistance between the aorta and the pulmonary artery. In cases where there is a very large left-to-right shunt at the ductal level, the large amount of pulmonary venous return will cause left atrial and left ventricular enlargement.

Natural History

The natural history of a patent arterial duct depends greatly on the size of the duct, the pulmonary vascular resistance, and the amount of flow from the aorta into the pulmonary artery. If the duct is quite small, there may be no murmur, and the diagnosis is only made "accidentally" on an echocardiogram. Whether or not those patients are at risk for endocarditis is controversial. Because the true incidence of a "silent ductus" is unknown, and the risk of endocarditis is very low, many pediatric cardiologists do not believe that the silent ductus requires therapy.

If the ductus is larger, the flow from the aorta into the pulmonary artery hits against the anterior wall of the pulmonary artery [1]. This rapid blood flow can cause a murmur in systole and diastole, often called a "machinery" murmur. Because this rapid flow can damage the endothelium of the pulmonary artery (the lining) this area is susceptible to bacterial deposition and subsequent growth, meaning endocarditis. For this reason, patients with an audible ductus should have the ductus closed.

Rarely, the ductus is large enough that the pressure transmitted into the pulmonary artery, along with the extra blood flow into the pulmonary artery results in pulmonary vascular disease. When the pulmonary arterial resistance reaches that of the systemic vascular resistance, the ductus can now shunt from the pulmonary artery into the aorta, otherwise known as right to left. In this situation the patient has "Eisenmeinger's syndrome". This is most frequently seen in patients with a predisposition for pulmonary vascular disease, such as patients with Down syndrome.

Surgical Options

Because of the risk of endocarditis, patients with an audible patent arterial duct should have closure of the ductus. This can be accomplished either in the catheterization laboratory, or in the operating room, depending upon the size of the duct and the local expertise. Either technique should provide a safe and effective way to completely close the duct, so that the patient is no longer at increased risk of bacterial endocarditis [2].

Auscultation

As with the physiology, the auscultation in a patient with a patent arterial duct depends on the size of the duct and the amount of flow from the aorta into the pulmonary artery. In patients with a very small duct, the physical examination should be normal, with normal precordial activity, a normal first and second heart sound, and no murmur. If the duct is moderate in size, the loud machinery systolic murmur may obscure both the first and the second heart sounds, as the flow from the aorta into the pulmonary artery occurs both in systole and diastole. Because of the large blood return to the left atrium, a diastolic rumble across the mitral valve is occasionally heard (see CD-ROM waveform). The peripheral pulses should be bounding, as the systolic pressure is normal or slightly elevated, and the diastolic pressure is low. If the patient has a large duct and pulmonary vascular disease (Eisenmeinger's syndrome) the precordial activity is normal, the first heart sound normal, and the second heart sound is loud and single, as the pressure in the pulmonary artery and aorta is equal. The pulses are normal, but depending on the amount of the right-to-left shunt, the patient may have cyanotic extremities (Tables 5.1, 5.2).

Table 5.1. Patent arterial duct

Precordial activity	Increased if there is a large amount of flow
First heart sound (S1)	May be obscured
Second heart sound (S2)	May be obscured
Systolic murmur	Harsh "machinery"
Grade	Grade 1–6
Location	Upper left sternal border
Diastolic murmur	Upper left sternal border
femoral pulses	Bounding

Table 5.2. What you hear on the CD-ROM

Patent ductus arteriosus	Upper right sternal border	Upper left sternal border	Lower left sternal border	Apex
First heart sound	Not audible	Not audible	Not audible	Not audible
Second heart sound	Single	Splits normally	Faint and single	Soft single sound
Systole	Grade 2/6 harsh murmur	Grade 3/6 harsh murmur	Grade 2/6 harsh	Grade 2/6 harsh murmur
Diastole	Grade 1/4 high pitched	Grade 3/4 high pitched	Grade 2/4 high pitched	Grade 2/4 high pitched

Subacute Bacterial Endocarditis Prophylaxis Recommendations (SBE)

According to the guidelines published by the American Heart Association in 2007, patients with a patent arterial defect do not require antibiotic prophylaxis at times of endocarditis risk [3].

In summary, persistent patency of the arterial duct is relatively rare. It causes a loud continuous murmur heard at the upper left sternal border, heard in both systole and diastole.

References

1. Bennhagen RG, Benson LN (2003) Silent and audible persistent ductus arteriosus: an angiographic study. Pediatr Cardiol 24(1):27–30

2. Ewert P (2005) Challenges encountered during closure of patent ductus arteriosus. Pediatr Cardiol 26(3):224–229

3. Wilson W, Taubert K, Gewitz M et al. (2007) Prevention of infective endocarditis. Guidelines from the American Heart Association. A Guideline From the American Heart Association Rheumatic Fever, Endocarditis, and Kawasaki Disease Committee, Council on Cardiovascular Disease in the Young, and the Council on Clinical Cardiology, Council on Cardiovascular Surgery and Anesthesia, and the Quality of Care and Outcomes Research Interdisciplinary Working Group 2007. Circulation April 19

Chapter 6
Aortic Stenosis

M.E. McConnell, *Pediatric Heart Sounds*,
DOI: 10.1007/978-1-84628-684-1_6, © Springer-Verlag London Limited 2008

Introduction

Stenosis of the aortic valve is a relatively common cardiac abnormality, accounting for 7.6% of congenital heart disease, with an
incidence of roughly 5 per 10,000 children [1].

Anatomy

The normal aortic valve has three leaflets that open completely with
ventricular systole, allowing blood to flow from the left ventricle to
the aorta without turbulence. Aortic stenosis can be at the subvalvar,
valvar, or supra valvar levels, with abnormalities of the valve itself
accounting for most of the cases. In patients with aortic valve
stenosis, the valve leaflets open incompletely, causing obstruction
between the left ventricle and the aorta (Fig. 6.1a, b).

In a recent study of aortic valves removed at the time of aortic
valve replacement for severe aortic stenosis, Roberts found that
54% had congenitally malformed valves. Of these malformations,
9% were unicuspid, and the remainder with abnormal valves was
bicuspid. Forty-five percent of their patients who had aortic valve
replacement had tricuspid aortic valves [2].

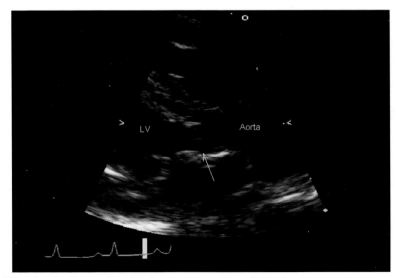

Fig. 6.1a. An abnormal aortic valve as seen on echocardiography

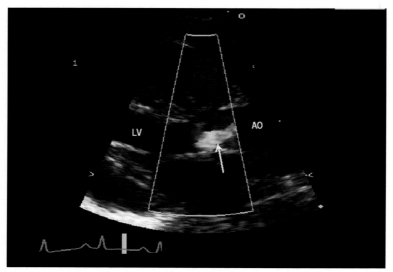

Fig. 6.1b. An echocardiogram of a child with aortic valve stenosis. *LV* left ventricle, *AO* aorta. The *arrow* points to the thick, stenotic aortic valve. The *yellow* and *blue* colors in the region of the aortic valve denote flow turbulence caused by the stenosis

Physiology

The physiology in a patient with aortic stenosis depends on the severity of the obstruction, the age of the patient, and the ventricular function. If the obstruction is severe, infants with aortic stenosis may be critically ill at birth, with poorly functioning left ventricles. The arterial duct may provide flow to the systemic circulation in these cases. This is because the aortic valve opens minimally, and the blood flow from the left ventricle to the aorta is inadequate. For the infant to have adequate blood flow into the aorta and subsequently to all the systemic organs, blood must circulate across the pulmonary valve, through the patent arterial duct, and into the aorta. In this way systemic cardiac output is maintained. Maintaining ductal patency with the administration of prostaglandin may be necessary until the patient can have a procedure to provide improved systemic blood flow. Patients with milder forms of aortic stenosis may show little or no outward signs of cardiac abnormalities. The obstruction may cause a loud murmur, but normal cardiac output can be maintained unless the patient puts significant stress on their cardiovascular system.

Natural History

The natural history of aortic valve stenosis depends on the severity of the left ventricular outflow tract obstruction. Unlike pulmonary valve stenosis, that is felt to be slowly progressive, if at all, patients with aortic valve stenosis often have worsening of the outflow tract obstruction [3]. This progressive obstruction may lead to symptoms of exercise intolerance, syncope, angina, and progressive dyspnea [4] Patients with bicuspid aortic valves are also at risk of developing dilatation of the ascending aorta. In the past, this dilatation was felt to be "post stenotic", meaning it was a consequence of the obstruction between the left ventricle and the aorta, and the subsequent rapid blood flow from the ventricle into the ascending aorta. Findings of dilated aortic roots in patients with bicuspid aortic valves and no significant obstruction bring this theory into question. The important point is that patients with an abnormal aortic valve can have an abnormal aorta as well, and these patients deserve lifelong cardiology follow up. Severe enlargement of the ascending aorta may result in aortic dissection or rupture, and intervention to replace a significantly dilated ascending aorta is often warranted.

Auscultatory Findings

The auscultatory findings in a patient with valvar aortic stenosis depend on the severity of the obstruction. With mildly abnormal aortic valves, the precordial activity would be normal, and there would not be a thrill palpable in the suprasternal notch. At the lower left sternal border, the first heart sound may sound like it has two parts to it, or that it splits. Actually this "splitting" is the clicking open of the abnormal aortic valve, and it is usually heard best at the apex. The first component of the split first heart sound is caused by the mitral and the tricuspid valves closing, and this is followed closely by the clicking open of the abnormal aortic valve. In contrast to the pulmonary valve ejection click, the aortic click does not vary with respiration. Following the aortic ejection click, a systolic murmur caused by blood coursing over the abnormal aortic valve should be heard at the upper sternal border, usually best on the right side. The murmur can range from grade 1 to 3/6 in the case of mild aortic stenosis (see CD-ROM waveform). The second heart sound should be normal. If the abnormal aortic valve leaks, the patient will have a diastolic murmur, heard best at the lower left sternal border.

In cases of more severe aortic stenosis, a thrill should be palpable at the suprasternal notch, or the upper right sternal border. The aortic click should still be heard at the apex. The murmur may be as loud as grade 6/6, meaning it can be heard with the stethoscope off of the chest altogether. The second heart sound is often narrowly split, as the abnormal aortic valve closes late, and at the same time as the pulmonic valve. The recording on the CD was taken from a patient with severe aortic stenosis. It has a loud click, heard at the apex, and a harsh, grade 5/6 systolic murmur loudest at the upper right sternal border. The second heart sound is narrowly split, due to the delayed aortic valve closure (Tables 6.1, 6.2).

Table 6.1 Aortic valve stenosis

Precordial activity	Possibly a thrill at the upper right sternal border and/or the suprasternal notch
First heart sound (S1)	Associated with a click at the apex that does not vary with respiration
Second heart sound (S2)	May be narrowly split
Systolic murmur	
Grade	Grade 1–6
Location	Right upper sternal border, often radiating to the neck and back
Diastolic murmur	None
Femoral pulses	Normal

Table 6.2. What you hear on the CD-ROM

Aortic valve stenosis	Upper right sternal border	Upper left sternal border	Lower left sternal border	Apex
First heart sound	Multiple because of a click	Multiple because of a click	Multiple because of a click	Multiple because of a click
Second heart sound	Single	Splits and varies	Splits and varies	Splits and varies
Systole	Grade 4/6 ejection	Grade 2/6 ejection	Grade 2/6 ejection	Grade 2/6 ejection
Diastole	No murmur	No murmur	No murmur	No murmur

Subacute Bacterial Endocarditis Prophylaxis Recommendations (SBE)

According to the guidelines published by the American Heart Association in 2007, patients with aortic stenosis do not require antibiotic prophylaxis at times of endocarditis risk, unless they have had a prior case of endocarditis [5].

Summary

Aortic valve disease is relatively common and can progress over the patients' lifetime. It is often associated with a click at the apex, which sounds like a "split first heart sound". Because of long-term complications of aortic valve disease, such as endocarditis, progressive obstruction to left ventricular outflow, and aortic root dilatation, diagnosis and lifelong cardiology follow up is important.

References

1. Samanek M, Slavik Z, Zborilova B, Hrobonova V, Voriskova M, Skovranek J (1989) Prevalence, treatment, and outcome of heart disease in live-born children: a prospective analysis of 91,823 live-born children. Pediatr Cardiol 10(4):205–211

2. Roberts WC, Ko JM (2005) Frequency by decades of unicuspid, bicuspid, and tricuspid aortic valves in adults having isolated aortic valve replacement for aortic stenosis, with or without associated aortic regurgitation. Circulation 111(7):920–925

3. Friedman WF, Modlinger J, Morgan J (1971) Serial hemodynamic observations in asymptomatic children with valvar aortic stenosis. Circulation 43:91

4. Hunter S (2002) Congenital anomalies of the aortic valve and left ventricular outflow tract. In: Anderson RH, Backer EJ et al (eds.) Paediatric cardiology. Churchill Livingstone, London, second edn pp 1481–1503

5. Wilson W, Taubert K, Gewitz M et al. (2007) Prevention of Infective Endocarditis. Guidelines From the American Heart Association. A Guideline From the American Heart Association Rheumatic Fever, Endocarditis, and Kawasaki Disease Committee, Council on Cardiovascular Disease in the Young, and the Council on Clinical Cardiology, Council on Cardiovascular Surgery and Anesthesia, and the Quality of Care and Outcomes Research Interdisciplinary Working Group 2007. Circulation April 19

Chapter 7
Pulmonary Stenosis

M.E. McConnell, *Pediatric Heart Sounds*,
DOI: 10.1007/978-1-84628-684-1_7, © Springer-Verlag London Limited 2008

Introduction

Stenosis of the pulmonary valve is a common form of congenital heart disease. One study estimates the incidence of congenital heart disease overall as 6.6/1,000 newborn infants. Of these children, 7.1% have pulmonary valve stenosis (0.46/1000) [1].

Anatomy

The pulmonary valve is a tri-leaflet structure that separates the right ventricular infundibulum from the pulmonary artery. Normally, the thin pliable leaflets of the pulmonary valve open with systole, and do not obstruct blood flow from the right ventricle to the pulmonary artery. In patients with pulmonary valve stenosis, the valve leaflets open incompletely, causing obstruction between the right ventricle and the pulmonary artery (Fig. 7.1).

Right ventricular outflow tract obstruction may also occur at the subvalvar level or the supravalvar level (see Fig. 7.2),

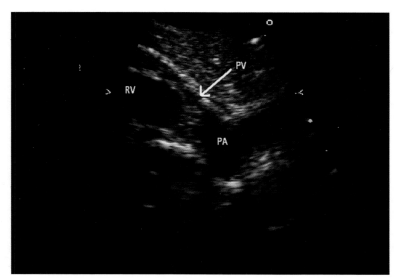

Fig. 7.1a. Long axis echocardiogram of a patient with an abnormal pulmonary valve

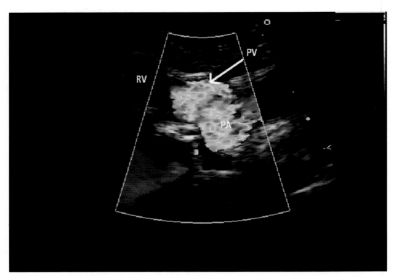

Fig. 7.1b. Color flow mapping across the same stenotic pulmonary valve. *RV* right ventricle, *PA* pulmonary artery, *PV* pulmonary valve. The *arrow* points to the thick, stenotic pulmonary valve leaflets, and the multiple colors are caused by the turbulent flow across the stenotic valve

but these lesions are much less common than valvar pulmonic stenosis [2].

Physiology

The physiology of the patient with pulmonary valve stenosis depends on the amount of stenosis, the pulmonary vascular resistance, and any associated defects in the heart. For a patient with mild stenosis, normal pulmonary vascular resistance, and no other cardiac abnormalities, there should be no significant physiologic consequences from the mildly stenotic pulmonary valve. The patient should not have a right to left or left to right shunt, should have normal cardiac output, and should have no symptoms related to the abnormal pulmonary valve. A newborn with severe pulmonary stenosis will have a great variability in physiology. For example, if the valve is severely stenotic, and very little blood can flow from the right ventricle to the pulmonary artery, the patient may require the presence of the

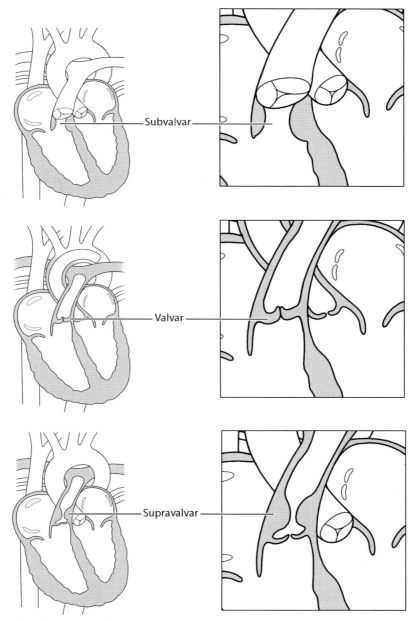

Fig. 7.2. Types of pulmonary stenosis. The obstruction between the right ventricle and the pulmonary artery can exist at the subvalvar, valvar, and supra valvar area. Often the obstruction is at a combination of the above locations

arterial duct and a patent atrial septum in order to have adequate cardiac output and adequate pulmonary blood flow.

The severely stenotic pulmonary valve would not allow adequate amounts of blood to leave the RV and go into the pulmonary artery. Therefore, the right atrial pressure will rise, and the deoxygenated blood will flow from the right atrium to the left atrium. This blood will then mix with the oxygenated blood returning from the pulmonary veins, and then flow through the mitral valve and into the left ventricle, where it will be pumped out of the aorta. If the arterial duct is open, some of the aortic blood will pass through the ductus and into the pulmonary artery. The newborn with severe pulmonary valve stenosis may therefore be cyanotic, because of the right to left flow of deoxygenated blood at the atrial level. The child may also be "ductal dependent" meaning that the blood through the arterial duct is necessary to provide adequate pulmonary blood flow to sustain life. In this situation, institution of medications that will maintain duct patency may be life saving.

Another example of the variable physiology in pulmonary valve stenosis is the infant with moderate-to-severe pulmonary valve stenosis and increased pulmonary vascular resistance shortly after birth. The infant may be asymptomatic, with a soft systolic murmur at the upper left sternal border, caused by flow across the stenotic pulmonary valve. Over the next few weeks, as the pulmonary vascular resistance drops, the obstruction between the RV and the pulmonary artery becomes more noticeable. This is because the murmur intensity is dependent on the change in pressure between the right ventricle and the pulmonary artery. In the newborn, the pulmonary artery pressure may be high, and therefore the difference in pressure between the right ventricle and the pulmonary artery will be low. This small difference between the right ventricular pressure and the pulmonary artery pressure at birth means that the murmur caused by flow across the stenotic pulmonary valve will be soft. As the pulmonary vascular resistance drops, the stenosis does not change, but the pressure difference between the right ventricle and the pulmonary artery may change significantly. Thus, a child thought to have mild pulmonary valve stenosis in the newborn period may have severe obstruction between the RV and PA by 2–3 months of life (see Fig. 7.3)

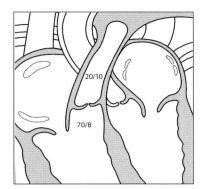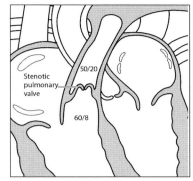

Fig. 7.3. The difference in measured obstruction or "pressure gradient" between the right ventricle and the pulmonary artery depending on the pulmonary artery pressure. In the left panel, the pulmonary artery pressure is low, and the "pressure gradient" (the difference between the systolic pressure in the right ventricle and the systolic pressure in the pulmonary artery) is 50 mmHg (70 mmHg – 20 mmHg = 50 mmHg). In the right panel, the pulmonary artery pressure is high, and therefore the gradient between the RV and PA is only 10 mmHg (60 – 50 mmHg). This can occur in newborn infants with severe right ventricular outflow tract obstruction who still have high pulmonary artery pressure

Natural History

The natural history of a patient with valvar pulmonic stenosis depends on the severity of the lesion. In patients with mild stenosis, exercise tolerance and life expectancy are near normal, and therefore no intervention should be contemplated for these patients. For patients with severe pulmonary valve stenosis, intervention to open the pulmonary valve, either with a balloon catheter or in the operating room may be life saving. In the first Natural History Study of Congenital Heart Defects (NHS), 592 patients with pulmonary stenosis were enrolled after catheterization, between 1958 and 1969. If the patient had mild pulmonary stenosis, defined as a gradient in the catheterization laboratory of <50 mmHg, the patients were managed medically. This group of patients had excellent long-term survival, and a less than 20% chance of requiring intervention on the right ventricular outflow tract. If the gradient was >50 mmHg (measured directly in the catheterization laboratory), most patients required intervention to enlarge the right ventricular outflow tract. Morbid events were uncommon in either the operated or unoperated patients with pulmonary stenosis, and the long-term life expectancy was identical to people without congenital heart disease. Patients who entered the study without cardiomegaly on CXR had no mortality during the study period, whereas patients with cardiomegaly who entered the study at more than 12 years of age had a 25-year survival rate of <80% [3]

In 1982 Kan et al. reported the first case of dilation of a stenotic pulmonary valve using a balloon catheter [4]. Since then, percutaneous dilatation of a stenotic pulmonary valve has become the treatment of choice for infants, children, and adults with right ventricular outflow tract obstruction at the level of the pulmonary valve. The long-term survival of patients treated with balloon dilatation is excellent. Although reintervention after an operation to open the pulmonary valve was rare, it is possible that the long-term effect of a leaking pulmonary valve will result in right ventricular dilatation and the need for pulmonary valve replacement in some patients [5]. Because of the benign natural history of mild pulmonary valve stenosis, and the fact that balloon dilatation of the pulmonary valve will often result in pulmonary valve insufficiency, some patients with mild pulmonary valve stenosis may not benefit in the long term from balloon dilatation of the mildly stenotic pulmonary valve, and should therefore be left alone. Endocarditis was very rare in patients with pulmonary valve stenosis. In fact there were no cases of endocarditis reported in the NHS study. The American Heart Association no longer recommends antibiotic prophylaxis at times of endocarditis risk for patients with pulmonic stenosis [6].

Auscultatory Findings

The physical examination of a patient with pulmonary valve stenosis depends greatly on the severity of the obstruction between the two ventricles, and the pulmonary artery pressure, as discussed above. For mild pulmonary stenosis, the precordial activity should be normal, and there will be no palpable thrill at the upper left sternal border (the pulmonary area). In patients with severe pulmonary stenosis, palpation of the precordium may reveal a left parasternal heave consistent with high right ventricular pressure. The flow across the stenotic pulmonary valve causes such turbulence that a thrill is felt in the left upper sternal border, over the pulmonic area. The thrill may also be palpable over the left side of the neck [7].

The abnormal sounds will be high pitched, and therefore heard best with the diaphragm of the stethoscope. Because the obstruction to blood flow is at the pulmonary valve level, the murmur will begin only after the pulmonary valve opens. The first heart sound is normal, but there is often a pulmonary ejection click caused by the opening of the abnormal pulmonary valve. The click is thought to be caused by the abnormal pulmonary valve clicking open, and therefore follows the first heart sound. The click of pulmonary valve stenosis sounds like "splitting" of the first heart sound. The mitral and tricuspid valves close, making the first sound. This is followed very rapidly (approximately 40 msec) [8] by the clicking open of the pulmonary valve. This splitting is best heard at the upper left sternal border, in the pulmonary area. Because the pulmonary valve leaflets move with inspiration, the valve leaflets "float" superiorly when the patient takes in a breath. This movement of the pulmonary valve makes the valve open from a different location, and therefore the pulmonary ejection sound often disappears with inspiration. Thus the click sounds like a split first heart sound that varies with respiration. The click can be so loud it is palpable, and the palpable click can disappear with the patient taking in a deep breath. On the CD-ROM recording, the pulmonary valve ejection sound is a loud "pop" heard intermittently at either the lower left sternal border, or the upper left sternal border. Listen carefully to the first heart sound until it is clear there is an "extra" sound that is not constant. This extra sound is the clicking open of the pulmonary valve. The second heart sound is caused by the closure of the abnormal pulmonary valve. In mild-to-moderate pulmonary valve stenosis, the abnormal pulmonic valve closes late, resulting in a split second heart sound. In patients with severe pulmonary valve stenosis, the pulmonary valve closure sound may be inaudible. The systolic murmur is caused by the flow of blood across the stenotic pulmonary valve, and causes a crescendo/decrescendo systolic murmur heard best at the upper left sternal border. The murmur does not change with respiration or position . In the case of severe obstruction between the right ventricle and the pulmonary artery, the murmur caused by the obstruction can obscure both the first and second heart sounds. In a young child, where the difference in the upper left sternal border and the lower left sternal border is small, a patient with severe pulmonary valve stenosis may be mistaken for a patient with a ventricular septal defect. Unless there is leakage of the pulmonary valve, there is no diastolic murmur (see Tables 7.1, 7.2)

Table 7.1. Pulmonary valve stenosis (moderate to severe)

Precordial activity	Possibly a thrill at the upper left sternal border and a left parasternal heave
First heart sound (S1)	Associated with a click that varies with respiration
Second heart sound (S2)	Widely split, and may be obscured
Systolic murmur	
Grade	Grade 3–6
Location	Left upper sternal border, often radiating to the axillae
Diastolic murmur	None
Femoral pulses	Normal

Table 7.2. What you hear on the CD-ROM

Pulmonary valve stenosis	Upper right sternal border	Upper left sternal border	Lower left sternal border	Apex
First heart sound	Multiple because of a click	Multiple because of a click	Multiple because of a click	Multiple because of a click
Second heart sound	Splits	Splits constantly because of the abnormal pulmonic valve	Splits	Splits
Systole	Grade 1/6 ejection	Grade 3/6 ejection	Grade 1/6 ejection	Grade 1/6 ejection
Diastole	No murmur	No murmur	No murmur	No murmur

Subacute Bacterial Endocarditis Prophylaxis Recommendations (SBE)

According to the guidelines published by the American Heart Association in 2007, patients with pulmonary valce stenosis do not require antibiotic prophylaxis at times of endocarditis risk, unless they have had a prior case of endocarditis [6].

In summary, pulmonary valve stenosis has a variable natural history depending on the severity of the obstruction. The physical examination features may include a left parasternal thrill, an ejection click that varies with respiration, a systolic murmur at the upper left sternal border, and a widely split second heart sound.

References

1. Samanek M, Slavik Z, Zborilova B, Hrobonova V, Voriskova M, Skovranek J (1989) Prevalence, treatment, and outcome of heart disease in live-born children: a prospective analysis of 91,823 liveborn children. Pediatr Cardiol 10:205–211

2. Kjellberg SR., Mannheimer E., Rudhe U, Jonsson B (1955) Diagnosis of congenital heart disease. Year Book Publishers, Chicago

3. Hayes CJ, Gersony WM, Driscoll DJ, Keane JF, Kidd L, O'Fallon WM, Pieroni DR, Wolfe RR, Weidman WH (1993) Second natural history study of congenital heart defects. Results of treatment of patients with pulmonary valvar stenosis. Circulation 87(2 Suppl):I28–I37

4. Kan JS, White RI Jr, Mitchell SE, Gardner TJ (1982) Percutaneous balloon valvuloplasty: a new method for treating congenital pulmonary-valve stenosis. [Case Reports. Journal article] New Engl J Med 307(9):540–542

5. Poon LK, Menahem S (2003) Pulmonary regurgitation after percutaneous balloon valvoplasty for isolated pulmonary valvar stenosis in childhood. Cardiol Young 13(5):444–450

6. Wilson W, Taubert K, Gewitz M et al. (2007) Prevention of Infective Endocarditis. Guidelines from the American Heart Association. A Guideline From the American Heart Association Rheumatic Fever, Endocarditis, and Kawasaki Disease Committee, Council on Cardiovascular Disease in the Young, and the Council on Clinical Cardiology, Council on Cardiovascular Surgery and Anesthesia, and the Quality of Care and Outcomes Research Interdisciplinary Working Group 2007. Circulation April 19

7. Levine SA, Harvey WP (1959) Clinical auscultation of the heart. W.B. Saunders, New York, pp 453–463

8. Waider W, Craige E (1975) First heart sound and ejection sounds. Echocardiographic and phonocardiographic correlation with valvular events. Am J Cardiol 35(3):346–356

Chapter 8
Mitral Valve Insufficiency

M.E. McConnell, *Pediatric Heart Sounds*,
DOI: 10.1007/978-1-84628-684-1_8, © Springer-Verlag London Limited 2008

Introduction

Isolated congenital abnormalities of the mitral valve are relatively rare, estimated at less than 0.1 per 1,000 live births [1]. The mitral valve may be damaged by rheumatic fever, or also may degenerate over time, resulting in mitral valve regurgitation.

Anatomy

The anatomy of a leaking mitral valve is variable, but for the sake of simplicity can be divided into two main abnormalities. The first, where the two leaflets of the mitral valve cannot completely close because there is a deformity in the valve, such as a cleft (see Fig. 8.1).

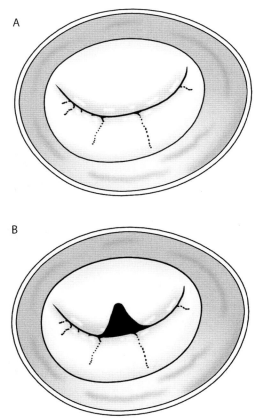

Fig. 8.1. A cleft mitral valve. **a** A normal mitral valve with a complete coaptation of the two leaflets. **b** An abnormal "cleft" mitral valve, with a wedge of tissue missing in the anterior leaflet of the mitral valve

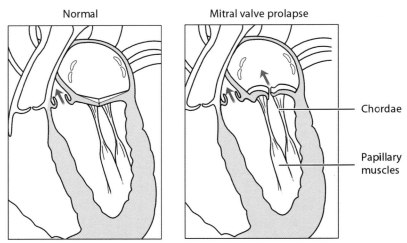

Fig. 8.2. Mitral valve prolapse. The abnormal mitral valve is seen in ventricular systole. The valve leaflets prolapse into the left atrium, and in late systole the leaflets cease to coapt, resulting in mitral valve regurgitation, depicted by the *right arrow*

A cleft is a defect in the mitral valve that acts like a hole. When the valve closes, blood is still able to pass through the hole in the valve from the left ventricle into the left atrium. The second type of mitral

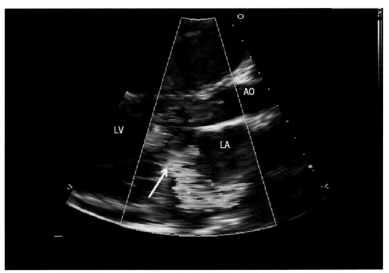

Fig. 8.3. Echocardiographic image in the parasternal long axis in a child with severe mitral valve regurgitation from a cleft mitral valve. *LA* left atrium, *LV* left ventricle, *AO* aorta. The *arrow* shows the blue plume of flow from the leaking mitral valve. The regurgitant jet flows toward the posterior left atrial wall, characteristic of a patient with a cleft anterior mitral valve leaflet

valve disease is mitral valve prolapse. In this condition, the leaflets of the mitral valve are long enough to coapt, but are too long and redundant, so that after the valve leaflets close, the valve leaflets pop open again. The valve now leaks, and blood is able to regurgitate from the left ventricle to the left atrium (see Figs. 8.2, 8.3).

Physiology

The physiology of mitral valve disease depends on the amount of regurgitation. In cases of mild mitral valve regurgitation from an abnormal mitral valve, the left atrium will be normal in size, and the left atrial pressure will be normal. This patient is unlikely to have symptoms related to the mitral valve regurgitation. With more severe leakage of the mitral valve, whether it is from mitral valve prolapse, or from a cleft mitral valve, the left atrial pressure will rise. This is because with each systole, the ventricle ejects a large amount of blood into the left atrium. The left atrial pressure rises, causing blood to back up into the pulmonary veins, and then the lungs. This high left atrial pressure can result in an elevated right ventricular pressure, and pulmonary hypertension as the right side of the heart works to force blood through the high pressure left atrium. Because forward flow through the pulmonary bed is impaired, patients with moderate-to-severe mitral valve regurgitation often have shortness of breath, especially with physical exertion.

Natural History

The natural history of mitral valve disease depends to a great extent on the severity and etiology of the abnormal mitral valve. For an isolated cleft valve, with mild regurgitation, the natural history should be normal. If there is more severe regurgitation, the patient might require surgery to repair, or even replace the abnormal mitral valve.

Surgical Options

The surgical options for patients with significant mitral valve regurgitation depend on the etiology of the regurgitation. If the valve has a cleft so that the leaflets are not able to completely close, surgery to repair the cleft is often quite successful. This surgery is usually quite safe, with an operative survival in good centers approaching 100%. If the valve is floppy and redundant, like in some patients with the Marfan syndrome, surgical repair of the valve is more difficult. In situations where the repaired valve is likely to degenerate in a short period of time, the valve should probably be replaced, not repaired.

Auscultatory Findings

The auscultatory findings in a patient with mitral valve regurgitation depend on the severity of the regurgitation, and also on whether the valve leaks as the leaflet closes (like in a patient with a cleft mitral valve) or if the valve leaks only after the prolapsing mitral valve pops open.

Mitral valve regurgitation from a cleft mitral valve

If the patient has a cleft in the mitral valve that leaks as the mitral valve closes, the patient will have a murmur that begins as the mitral valve closes, therefore obscuring the first heart sound. If the regurgitation is mild, the left atrial pressure is normal, and the pulmonary artery pressure is likewise normal. The second heart sound will therefore be normal, and will split with respiration. If the valve leaks severely, the left atrial pressure will be high, and therefore the pulmonary artery pressure will also be high. This high pulmonary artery pressure will cause a loud second heart sound, as the pulmonary valve and the aortic valve are forced closed by similar high pressures. The systolic murmur caused by the leaking mitral valve is a harsh sound, heard best at the apex. If the regurgitation is severe, there will be a diastolic murmur caused by the large volume of blood flowing from the left atrium into the left ventricle across the mitral valve. This diastolic rumbling sound is low pitched, and often difficult to appreciate. It has been described as an "absence of silence", and can be heard best on the CD in the patient with an ASD. The mitral valve regurgitation recording is not of a large enough volume to cause a diastolic murmur. If it was present, the diastolic rumble would be heard best with the bell of the stethoscope, placed at the apex of the left ventricle, and pressed down so that the skin beneath the mitral valve is tight, and the bell

Table 8.1. Mitral valve regurgitation from a cleft mitral valve

Mitral valve regurgitation	Cleft mitral valve
Precordial activity	Increased if there is a large amount of regurgitation
First heart sound (S1)	Obscured
Second heart sound (S2)	May be loud if there is a large amount of regurgitation
Systolic murmur	
Grade	Grade 1–6
Location	Apex (mitral area)
Diastolic murmur	Possible diastolic rumble across the mitral valve
femoral pulses	Normal

acts like a diaphragm. The high-frequency sounds are then best heard. Then you should lighten up on the bell, and let it act more like a bell, where it will transmit the low-frequency sounds. Then, in cases where there is a large volume of blood flowing from the LA to the LV in diastole, you should hear a rumbling sound in diastole. This implies that the mitral valve regurgitation is severe (Table 8.1).

Mitral valve regurgitation from a prolapsing mitral valve

Mitral valve regurgitation from a prolapsing mitral valve causes a physical examination that may be quite different from the examination in someone with a cleft mitral valve. If there is minimal mitral valve regurgitation the precordial activity will be normal. In classic mitral valve prolapse, the mitral valve closure causes a normal first heart sound. After the mitral valve closes, the valve pops superiorly into the left atrium, causing a click. After the valve clicks, the leaflets may open, causing mitral valve regurgitation. The murmur can occasionally have a strange, "honking" type quality. If the mitral valve leakage is mild, there will be normal left atrial pressure, and therefore a normal second heart sound. In the case of minimal mitral valve regurgitation, there will be no diastolic rumble. If the mitral valve prolapse results in severe mitral valve regurgitation, the patient may have a loud second heart sound, as well as a diastolic rumble across the mitral valve [2] (Tables 8.2, 8.3).

Table 8.2. Mitral valve regurgitation from mitral valve prolapse

Mitral valve regurgitation	Mitral valve prolapse
Precordial activity	Increased if there is a large amount of regurgitation
First heart sound (S1)	Normal followed by a late systolic click
Second heart sound (S2)	May be loud if there is a large amount of regurgitation
Systolic murmur	
Grade	Grade 1–6
Location	Apex (mitral area)
Diastolic murmur	Possible diastolic rumble across the mitral valve
Femoral pulses	Normal

Table 8.3. What you hear on the CD-ROM

Mitral valve regurgitation	Upper right sternal border	Upper left sternal border	Lower left sternal border	Apex
First heart sound	Not audible	Not audible	Not audible	Not audible
Second heart sound	Variably split	Variably split	Variably split	Faint and single
Systole	Grade 2/6 blowing murmur	Grade 2/6 blowing murmur	Grade 2/6 blowing murmur	Grade 2 to 3/6blowing murmur
Diastole	No murmur	No murmur	No murmur	No murmur

Subacute Bacterial Endocarditis Prophylaxis Recommendations (SBE)

According to the guidelines published by the American Heart Association in 2007, patients with mitral valve regurgitation do not require antibiotic prophylaxis at times of endocarditis risk, unless they have had a prior case of endocarditis [3].

In summary, murmurs of mitral valve regurgitation may or may not obscure the first heart sound, depending on when the valve begins to leak. If there is a large amount of regurgitation, the precordial activity will be increased, the second heart sound will be accentuated, and there will be a diastolic rumble across the mitral valve.

References

1. Samanek M, Slavik Z, Zborilova B, Hrobonova V, Voriskova M, Skovranek J (1989) Prevalence, treatment, and outcome of heart disease in live-born children: a prospective analysis of 91,823 live-born children. Pediatr Cardiol 10(4):205–211

2. Smallhorn J, Macartney FJ (2002). In: Anderson RH et al. (eds) Mitral valve anomalies and supravalvar mitral ring. Paediatric cardiology, second edn. Churchill Livingstone, London, pp 1135–1175

3. Wilson W, Taubert K, Gewitz M et al. (2007) Prevention of Infective Endocarditis. Guidelines from the American Heart Association. A Guideline From the American Heart Association Rheumatic Fever, Endocarditis, and Kawasaki Disease Committee, Council on Cardiovascular Disease in the Young, and the Council on Clinical Cardiology, Council on Cardiovascular Surgery and Anesthesia, and the Quality of Care and Outcomes Research Interdisciplinary Working Group 2007. Circulation April 19

Chapter 9
Tetralogy of Fallot

M.E. McConnell, *Pediatric Heart Sounds*,
DOI: 10.1007/978-1-84628-684-1_9, © Springer-Verlag London Limited 2008

Incidence

Tetralogy of Fallot is a relatively common form of congenital heart disease, and is seen in roughly 2–3 per 10,000 infants [1]. Because therapy for this disorder is usually successful, there are many adults with tetralogy of Fallot, and in some countries, there are more adults with the condition than children.

Anatomy

In 1888, Dr. Fallot described the cardiac anatomy of a patient with cyanosis who had a ventricular septal defect, an aorta that originated from both the right and left ventricles, obstruction between the right ventricle and the pulmonary artery, and a hypertrophied right ventricle (Fig. 9.1)

Although this anatomic combination had been described as early as the seventeenth century, it was Fallot's description that gave the eponym to this common form of cyanotic congenital heart disease [2]. The obstruction to blood flow from the right ventricle to the pulmonary artery may be at the pulmonary valve annulus, the sub-pulmonary area or the supra valvar area. Often, the obstruction from the right ventricle to the pulmonary artery is at all three levels.

Physiology

The physiology of a patient with tetralogy of Fallot is quite variable, depending on the amount of pulmonary blood flow. This is true for many forms of cyanotic congenital heart disease, and this is the reason that tetralogy of Fallot is used on the CD-ROM as an example of cyanotic heart disease. For example, in the situation where there is minimal obstruction between the right ventricle and the pulmonary artery, the ventricular septal defect will be the predominant pathologic feature, and the pulmonary blood flow will be increased. In this situation, the patient will not have cyanosis, and if there is too much pulmonary blood flow the patient may even exhibit signs of congestive heart failure, just like a patient with a large isolated ventricular septal defect. These patients may still have an overriding aorta, obstruction between the right ventricle and the pulmonary artery (albeit mild) and a hypertrophied right ventricle; so

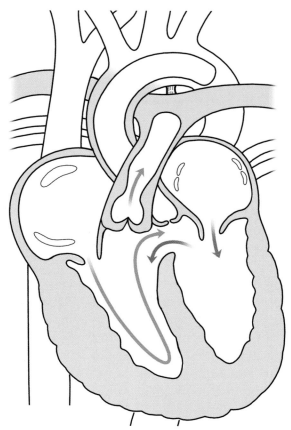

Fig. 9.1. Schematic representation of a patient with tetralogy of Fallot. Note the large ventricular septal defect, the aorta that can get blood flow from either the left or the right ventricle, the obstruction between the right ventricle and the pulmonary artery, and the thick right ventricle

technically they have tetralogy of Fallot. But their physiology is very different from the classic cases, and often these children will require early surgical intervention because of excessive pulmonary blood flow. These patients with tetralogy of Fallot and large left-to-right shunts are often referred to as "pink tets". In a more typical case of tetralogy of Fallot, the obstruction between the right ventricle and the pulmonary artery is moderate to severe. In this situation some of the blood leaving the right ventricle may flow into the aorta. Because this right ventricular blood is non-oxygenated blood, the blue blood within the aorta will cause cyanosis. It is important to note that the obstruction between the right ventricle and the pulmonary artery can change rapidly. This is particularly problematic if the obstruction is in the sub-pulmonary area, also known as the infundibulum (Figs. 9.2, 9.3).

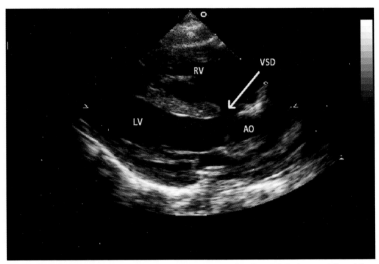

Fig. 9.2. Echocardiogram of an infant with tetralogy of Fallot. *LV* left ventricle, *AO* aorta, *RV* right ventricle. The *arrow* points to the large ventricular septal defect (VSD). Note also that the right ventricle wall is as thick as the left ventricular wall

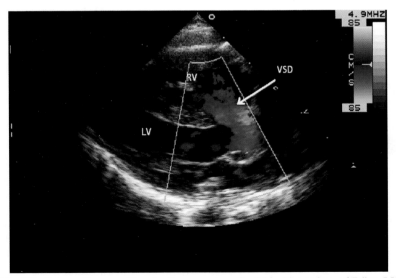

Fig. 9.3. Echocardiogram with color flow mapping of a child with tetralogy of Fallot. *LV* left ventricle, *RV* right ventricle, *VSD* ventricular septal defect. Note the *blue color*, denoting flow from the RV into the aorta

At times, especially if the child is dehydrated, the distance between the muscular walls of the infundibulum gets closer together, causing increased obstruction between the right ventricle and the pulmonary artery. When this happens, the pulmonary blood flow decreases, and the cyanosis worsens. This is also known as a tetralogy or "tet" spell. During a "tet" spell, calming the infant is important. In addition, during a tet spell, pushing the infant's knees into their chest will increase the systemic vascular resistance, and force more blood into the pulmonary circulation. This is why unoperated children with tetralogy of Fallot may "squat". This position effectively cuts off the femoral arterial blood flow, and increases the pulmonary blood flow. Patients with a ventricular septal defect and pulmonary stenosis have their physiology governed by the amount of pulmonary blood flow. This physiology is important in other forms of congenital heart disease as well. Examples include tricuspid atresia and single ventricles in which the amount of pulmonary blood flow regulates the amount and type of symptoms, just as it does in patients with tetralogy of Fallot.

Natural History

Because of operations to palliate patients with tetralogy of Fallot were first performed in the 1940s, and operations to correct the anatomical abnormalities were performed in the 1950s, in many countries, the "natural history" of tetralogy of Fallot is no longer applicable. The most recent estimate, however, suggests that without surgical intervention, at least 90% of patients with tetralogy of Fallot will die by 25 years of age [3]. Fortunately, with modern surgical techniques, most patients with uncomplicated tetralogy of Fallot can do very well. Long-term survival depends to a great extent on the quality of the pulmonary arteries preoperatively. if the pulmonary arteries are normal in size, in the current era, survival should be near that of the normal population. If the pulmonary arteries are small, or have multiple obstructions within them, the outlook may be much worse than the normal population. Twenty-five-year survival rates for patients with tetralogy of Fallot exceed 90% [4].

Surgical Options

Surgery for patients with tetralogy of Fallot involves closing the ventricular septal defect and opening the obstruction between the right ventricle and the pulmonary artery. The timing of this intervention varies from center to center, but should be safely performed at almost any age in the current era. In situations where the pulmonary arteries are small, or if the child is so small that complete correction is felt to be dangerous, a shunt is sometimes performed. The shunt operation connects the systemic arterial circulation to the pulmonary circulation, usually via a prosthetic tube. Post-operatively, some of the blood leaving the heart into the aorta is able to flow through the shunt, and therefore into the pulmonary artery, bypassing the obstruction between the right ventricle and the pulmonary artery. This shunt is named after the surgeon and pediatric cardiologist who participated in the initial surgical work, Drs. Blalock and Taussig. Additional credit is also due to Dr. Vivien Thomas, who was integral in the research leading to the first successful palliation of cyanotic congenital heart disease [5]. During the complete repair of tetralogy of Fallot, the surgeon attempts to open the right ventricle to pulmonary artery communication by removing the muscular tissue beneath the pulmonary valve. Often, the pulmonary valve annulus is significantly smaller than the aortic valve annulus. In order to make the outflow area from each ventricle similar in size, the surgeons often place an incision across the pulmonary valve annulus, and then sew a patch in the incision to widen the area (Fig. 9.4).

The significance of this operative technique is that the patient leaves the operating room without a functional pulmonary valve, and therefore will eventually have free pulmonary valve insufficiency. This situation will require replacement of a pulmonary valve in the distant future, often 15–30 years after the initial surgery.

Auscultatory Findings

The physical examination findings in a patient with tetralogy of Fallot vary widely, just like the physiology. When there is a moderate amount of obstruction from the right ventricle to the pulmonary artery, the patient should have normal precordial activity. Depending on the amount of blood flowing from the right ventricle into the

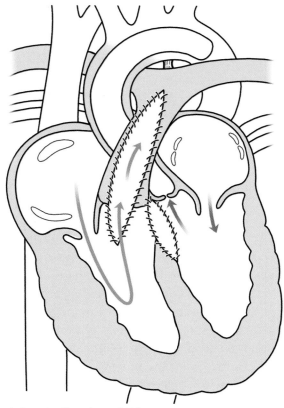

Fig. 9.4. Surgical repair of tetralogy of Fallot. Note the closure of the ventricular septal defect, as well as the widening of the right ventricular outflow tract. This widening results in a dysfunctional pulmonary valve. The pulmonary valve will eventually need to be replaced in almost all patients with repaired tetralogy of Fallot

aorta (right-to-left shunting), the patient will have a variable amount of cyanosis. The first heart sound may be obscured, but often a pulmonary ejection click is audible at the upper left sternal border. The second heart sound is often single, because the closure sound of the smaller pulmonary valve is inaudible. The murmur is caused by blood flowing from the high-pressure right ventricle into the low-pressure pulmonary artery, and can vary from a grade 2 to 3/6 ejection murmur, to a grade 6/6 harsh systolic murmur that is so loud it obscures all other heart sounds. When the obstruction between the right ventricle and the pulmonary artery is in the muscular tissue between the right ventricle and the pulmonary artery (the infundibulum) the physical examination can vary from minute to

Table 9.1. Tetralogy of fallot

Precordial activity	Normal
First heart sound (S1)	May be normal, may be associated with a click, or obscured if the murmur is very loud
Second heart sound (S2)	Usually single
Systolic murmur	
Grade	Grade 1–6
Location	Upper left sternal border
Diastolic murmur	None
Femoral pulses	Normal

Table 9.2. What you hear on the CD-ROM

Tetralogy of fallot	Upper right sternal border	Upper left sternal border	Lower left sternal border	Apex
First heart sound	Not audible	Not audible	Not audible	Not audible
Second heart sound	Obscured	Obscured	Faint single sound	Obscured
Systole	Grade 2/ 6 harsh murmur	Grade 3/ 6 harsh murmur	Grade 2/ 6 harsh	Grade 1/ 6 harsh
Diastole	no murmur	no murmur	no murmur	No murmur

minute in the same patient. This variability depends on the amount of blood flow going into the lungs. For example, if there is moderate obstruction, the physical examination will be as described above. If the patient's obstruction worsens, there may be a normal first heart sound, only a soft systolic murmur at the upper left sternal border, and a single second heart sound (Tables 9.1, 9.2).

Subacute Bacterial Endocarditis Prophylaxis Recommendations (SBE)

According to the guidelines published by the American Heart Association in 2007, patients with tetralogy of Fallot do require antibiotic prophylaxis at times of endocarditis risk, because they have cyanotic heart disease. Six months after they have been repaired, the patients no longer require antibiotic prophylaxis at times of endocarditis risk, unless they have a residual ventricular septal defect that jets against prosthetic patch material, or if they have a prosthetic valve. They will also require endocarditis prophylaxis if they have had a prior case of endocarditis [6].

In summary, tetralogy of Fallot is relatively common, and is an excellent example to help understand cyanotic congenital heart disease. Aucsultatory findings, as well as the amount of cyanosis vary widely, and depend on the severity of the obstruction between the right ventricle and the pulmonary artery.

References

1. Samanek M, Slavik Z, Zborilova B, Hrobonova V, Voriskova M, Skovranek J (1989) Prevalence, treatment, and outcome of heart disease in live-born children: a prospective analysis of 91,823 live-born children. Pediatr Cardiol 10(4):205–211

2. Fallot A (1888) Contribution a l'anatomie pathologique de la maladie bleue (cyanose cardiaque). Marseille, Barlatier-Feissat

3. Rygg IH, Olesen K, Boesen I (1971) The life history of tetralogy of Fallot. Dan Med Bull 18(Suppl 2):25–30

4. Pokorski RJ (2000)Long-term survival after repair of tetralogy of Fallot.J Insurance Med 32(2):89–92

5. Brogan TV, Alfieris GM (2003) Has the time come to rename the Blalock-Taussig shunt? Pediatr Crit Care Med 4(4):450–453

6. Wilson W, Taubert K, Gewitz M et al. (2007) Prevention of Infective Endocarditis. Guidelines from the American Heart Association. A Guideline From the American Heart Association Rheumatic Fever, Endocarditis, and Kawasaki Disease Committee, Council on Cardiovascular Disease in the Young, and the Council on Clinical Cardiology, Council on Cardiovascular Surgery and Anesthesia, and the Quality of Care and Outcomes Research Interdisciplinary Working Group 2007. Circulation April 19

Index

System Requirements

Windows XP operating system or newer, CD-ROM or DVD drive, 16-bit sound, speakers or headphones, a subwoofer speaker is recommended to hear low frequency sounds, and 800 x 600 screen resolution or higher, with at least 256 colors.

Instructions

- Insert CD-ROM into drive

- The program should launch automatically after your screen becomes dark. If a dialog box appears asking to run Ped Heart Sounds 2008.exe, indicate that you wish to run the program.

- If program does not launch, click on the **Start** button, then **My Computer** (**Computer** if using Vista). Double click on the CD drive containing Pediatric Heart Sounds.

- Once the program is running you should hear music playing. If you do not hear music, check your computer volume and mute settings.

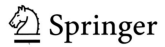

Printed in the United States of America

System Requirements

Windows XP operating system or newer, CD-ROM or DVD drive, 16-bit sound, speakers or headphones, a subwoofer speaker is recommended to hear low frequency sounds, and 800 x 600 screen resolution or higher, with at least 256 colors.

Instructions

- Insert CD-ROM into drive

- The program should launch automatically after your screen becomes dark. If a dialog box appears asking to run Ped Heart Sounds 2008.exe, indicate that you wish to run the program.

- If program does not launch, click on the **Start** button, then **My Computer** (**Computer** if using Vista). Double click on the CD drive containing Pediatric Heart Sounds.

- Once the program is running you should hear music playing. If you do not hear music, check your computer volume and mute settings.

Springer